AMERICAN ENVIRONMENTAL STUDIES

*The Uses
and
Abuses of Air*

JOHN H. GRISCOM

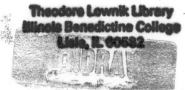
ARNO &
THE NEW YORK TIMES

Collection Created and Selected
by CHARLES GREGG of Gregg Press

Reprint Edition 1970 by Arno Press Inc.

Reprinted from a copy in
The Columbia University Library

LC# 79-125743
ISBN 0-405-02668-4

American Environmental Studies
ISBN for complete set: 0-405-02650-1

Manufactured in the United States of America

THE

USES AND ABUSES OF AIR:

SHOWING

ITS INFLUENCE IN SUSTAINING LIFE,

AND

PRODUCING DISEASE;

WITH REMARKS ON THE

VENTILATION OF HOUSES,

AND THE

BEST METHODS OF SECURING A PURE AND WHOLESOME
ATMOSPHERE INSIDE OF DWELLINGS, CHURCHES,
COURT-ROOMS, WORKSHOPS, AND BUILDINGS
OF ALL KINDS.

BY JOHN H. GRISCOM, M. D.,

PHYSICIAN OF THE NEW YORK HOSPITAL, FELLOW OF THE COLLEGE
OF PHYSICIANS AND SURGEONS, ETC.

SECOND EDITION.

NEW YORK:
J. S. REDFIELD, CLINTON HALL,
CORNER OF NASSAU AND BEEKMAN STREETS.

1850.

STEREOTYPED BY C. C. SAVAGE,
13 Chambers Street, N. Y.

THE USES AND ABUSES OF AIR.

CHAPTER I.

Health the greatest Earthly Desideratum.—Does not receive the most intelligent Attention.—Systems of Dietaries.—Croton Water.—Air neglected in Houses.—Relations of our Bodies to Food and Air.—One easy and the other difficult of Attainment.—Food often fails, Air never.

Though self-preservation is generally regarded as the mainspring of human action, and the first principle of our nature, it can not be denied that it is very often blind, with regard to the object it contemplates. Reason may often misguide, and ignorance deceive, no matter how cultivated the mind may be; but it is lamentable to see enlightened people, in this enlightened age, neglecting to study, nay, regarding with the coldest and most apathetic indifference, a subject, easy of comprehension, and one intimately connected with the physical, moral, and intellectual conditions of society; and, in fact, with the health, life, and happiness, of the human race. Health seems to be the *summum bonum*, the highest terrestrial aim, of both rich and poor; is esteemed the climax of all earthly blessings; and when lost, generally speaking, no consideration seems too great, no reward too high, for its restoration. Accordingly, we should expect, that as bad health is the result of a derangement of one or more of the vital functions, whether of *digestion, circulation, respiration,* or any other, and that, as these functions are mutually dependent, and co-existent, in the economy of life—the suspension of any given one being followed by a suspension of all the oth-ers—I say, we should expect that *all* these functions would be most assiduously administered to, and the most unrestricted encouragement given to their exercise Un-fortunately, such is not the case—for it too often hap-pens, that while one function, comfort, or convenience of life, has received due and even extravagant attention (as is instanced in the fashionable follies of dress), others, of equal or greater importance, are lightly regarded, or totally neglected.

For example, altogether irrespective of the subject of *clothing*, which engrosses so much attention in all civ-ilized nations—how many lectures have been delivered and books written, by eminent men, on the different sys-tems of dietetics, which have all been listened to, or carefully perused, and acted upon, by all classes in the community ! How ably, and eloquently, have the differ-ent articles of food been canvassed, analyzed, and classi-fied, according to their different degrees of nutrition or digestibility ! Even rival systems of *dietaries* have sprung up, and the advocates of each have not, in some instances, hesitated to indulge in the warmest discussions, and the most narrow-minded professional jealousy. Two sects, in particular, have made themselves conspicuous—the one advocating the necessity of eating animal food, the other averring that it is " rank poison," and that slaugh-tering dumb beasts for food, is an offence in the sight of Heaven ; while Grahamism is still studied and practised by a select few, with almost religious zeal, — and the Bi-ble is, as usual, appealed to, and quoted in defence of both opinions. Again, to show what prodigious labor—labor more than herculean—and disregarded expense, will be bestowed upon the comforts and health of a single community, in regard to the matter of drink alone, let us contemplate, for a moment, the introduction of the Croton water into the city of New York. It is enough to say, that nearly $15,000,000 have been expended on this project, and it may be added, judiciously expended. Now, an intelligent stranger, coming into town, would, after being made aware of these facts, naturally admire the enlightened and well-directed efforts for the dietetic amelioration of the people, and applaud the enterprise and sagacity that decoyed the refreshing current into every street and lane of our thirsty city; but he would as naturally ask, What provision have you made to introduce into your public schools, workshops, jails, churches, benevolent institutions, and, above all, the humble dwellings of the poor, that life-giving, ethereal, and invisible fluid, without which food and water of any and every kind, are as useless for the purposes of nourishment, as the clay or sand? The question is a leading one, and the answer anticipated.

The relations of our bodies to the food which sustains them, are such, that when there is a necessity for an additional supply of it, nature has implanted within us certain *sensations, which indicate that necessity.* These sensations are painful, distressing, urgent, and of such a peculiar character, as at once to point to the means of relief. But our aliment is so placed, that we must *go in search of it.* It is not furnished immediately at our hands, and in such profusion that we can stand still and let it drop into our mouths; but we must employ the faculties of memory, judgment, and sight; we must exert our muscles to labor, our forethought, our knowledge of the seasons — of growth and decay — as well as our experience of the varieties adapted to the various conditions of the body, at different periods of the year, and hours of the day. And even with all these faculties in full

1*

vigor, and with the demands of nature pressing with
unwonted force upon our suffering bodies, nature will
sometimes withhold its supplies ; the soil will sometimes
cease to yield its fruits, which no art can supply before
thousands die by famine.

But how different is it with the atmosphere ! Except
under circumstances attending its total or near exclusion
from us (which are always accidental and very rare), we
have no well-defined and unerring sensations, to indicate
a necessity for air.   To denote the want of this element,
there is no sensation corresponding to those of hunger
or thirst, nor does the sense of taste enable us to detect
its impurities.   The atmosphere of a room, or even of
open space, may be deteriorated to a degree highly
injurious to health ; *yet we may be insensible to the fact.*
Upon going suddenly, from the open pure air, into an
impure atmosphere, we may indeed perceive, by some
disagreeable odor, that it is not proper to be breathed ;
but if its impurities have arisen while we have been
immersed in it, not only, as has been said, may we be
insensible thereto, but the impurity itself may have so
operated upon our faculties and sensations, as to have
benumbed them, and thus increased the danger.

But when was a deficient supply of air ever known,
except through the agency of man himself, in his folly
and ignorance ?   Providence has furnished us with an
ocean of it, fifty miles deep, and placed us at the bottom,
where its pressure enables us to obtain it in exhaustless
profusion, and perfect purity.   By the exercise of a certain corporeal function, which is carried on without our
notice or aid, it flows, surely and steadily, deep into the
body ; and so arranged are the functions, that it requires
more than one's ordinary physical strength, permanently
to arrest its flowing in.

To the helpless infant, both food and air are furnished

without its aid: but how differently! To be supplied with food, its cries must reach the ear of its mother, who must, herself, be supplied from other sources; while as to the air, without a care or a thought, without labor or sensation, the little animal instinctively expands its chest, and lives.

But the relations of the food and air to our bodies, which they conjointly support, and the true estimation in which they should be held, in regard to the attention necessary for their better adaptation to their important purposes, will be better appreciated by a more detailed comparison of them, in connexion with the manner in which they perform their parts, in giving sustenance and life. This will be done in the next chapter.

CHAPTER II.

Relative Importance of Food and Air.—Nature and Number of the Changes each undergoes.—Power of the System to separate Impurities from each.—Length of Time an Animal may live without either.—Digestion.—Respiration.—Each described.—Their Peculiarities.—Persons who breathe Impure Air, can not appreciate Pure Air so well.—Air necessary to Digestion.—Respiration the last Act of Digestion.—Surfeiting, common with Food, impossible with Air.

THE relative importance to the animal system, of the two principal sources of its support—viz: *the food it consumes,* and *the air it inhales*—may be determined upon the following points of comparison:—

First. The nature and number of the changes which each undergoes before being fitted to nourish the body; and the length of time, after each is received into the system, before it discharges its office.

Second. The power of the system to separate the impurities they may contain, and appropriate the good to its nourishment and support.

Third. The length of time that an animal may live without any addition of either respectively.

In order to appreciate, properly, the importance of these two sources of animal life and vigor, it is necessary to understand something of the functions by which each performs its part, and to be able to trace both, from the moment of their entrance into the interior of the body, to their ultimate destination.

The function by which all the food, solid and liquid, is made to nourish the animal body, is called *digestion.*

That by which atmospheric air is introduced into the chest, and enabled to act upon the system, is called *respiration.*

In considering the points of comparison just mentioned, we will, *first*, trace the course which the food takes, and observe the various changes wrought upon it, ere it enters the blood-vessels as nutrient matter.

After being masticated and mixed with saliva, it is swallowed and enters the stomach. In this organ it undergoes the first great change, being operated upon by the gastric juice, a powerful solvent, by which its whole character is reduced, from a heterogeneous mass of materials, to a homogeneous substance of a cream color — a semi-fluid consistence — and giving little or no trace of the different substances of which it was originally composed.

Animal and vegetable solids are all altered and reduced to this one substance, which has the name of *chyme.* This process being completed, the food in this new form is passed from the stomach into another organ, called the *duodenum*, or second stomach.

It is there mingled with other fluids, the principal of which is the *bile* (formed by the liver). These have the property of still further altering its chemical character; and the change which is here to be especially noted, is, that the impure and innutritious portion is partially separated from that which is fitted to nourish the body.

Passing onward from this organ, it enters the upper portion of the intestinal canal, the surface of which is studded with the mouths of innumerable capillary vessels, called lacteals.* In this situation, a complete separation of the nutritious from the innutritous parts of the food is made. The innutritious is carried onward and discharged from the body; while the pure, nutritious

* So called from the milky color of their contents.

part, called *chyle*, is absorbed by the lacteals, and transmitted from the intestines into a series of glands in the
same vicinity, where it undergoes a still further change.
This effected, it is conveyed upward from the abdomen,
by means of a duct, called (from its situation in the
chest, or thorax) the thoracic duct, which terminates in
a large vein, carrying a current of blood directly to the
heart. The substance thus conveyed by the thoracic
duct into the current of blood, and which mingles with,
and becomes a part of, the blood, is the purely nutritious
portion of the food, separated entirely from the useless,
or innutritious.

From even this cursory description, we see, that to
obtain this end, and to avoid the dangers that would follow the introduction of the crude food directly into the
circulation, a *long and manifold process*, having several
distinct steps, and employing a number of separate and
complicated organs, is required; and that, even then,
the food is not completely changed into blood, but is yet
only *chyle*.

The time occupied in thus preparing the food for
nutrition, varies with different articles of diet; but
probably is never less than two, and in many instances
extends to six or eight hours, before the completion of
the process. Fresh supplies of food are required not
more than three times, and frequently only twice, a-day.
But how different is it with the atmosphere in all these
particulars! It is no sooner inhaled than its work is
begun; and so rapid is its agency upon the blood, that
the inhalation of pure air is followed, almost immediately,
by the exhalation of the same air degenerated. *Twenty
times in a minute*, the blood requires an additional supply of oxygen, without which the whole body suffers.

Second. We observe that the digestive apparatus possesses the highly valuable, and very necessary, power of

separating the nutritious from the innutritious part of the food.

This is one of its most striking peculiarities. No such power of discrimination, however, is given to the process of respiration. The action of the gases inhaled, upon the blood circulating through the lungs, is direct, immediate, and positive. If an innocuous gas is taken in with the air, the lungs have no power of separating them; nor, if it be a poisonous gas, is there any power to deprive it of its injurious properties: but, for good or for evil, all that enters the lungs acts instantly upon the blood, according to its peculiar properties.

Moreover, the stomach has the power of rendering wholesome, substances which, under other circumstances, would prove prejudicial or even poisonous.

Ex. gr. Carbonic acid gas taken into the lungs in its purity causes speedy death, but may be swallowed in its pure form combined with water (soda or mineral water), with not only a harmless, but refreshing and invigorating effect.

Third. As regards the length of time that a person may exist without any additional food, it is believed to be about three weeks at the longest. Recovery at the end of this time may not be possible; but still, life may be continued this length of time, at the last burning more and more feebly in its socket.*

On the other hand, exclusion of atmospheric air from the lungs for the space of *three minutes*, will generally cause the death of the individual. Restorative opera-

---

* A case came to the knowledge of the writer, in 1843, of a woman, who, believing in the "Millerite" doctrine, was stricken with remorse at some serious misconduct; and, under the impression that her sin would be increased by partaking of any of the pleasures of life, refused utterly to eat or drink, and literally starved to death under the delusion. No means could induce her to taste anything, until so reduced in strength, force accomplished what her will denied: but unavailingly. She lived about three weeks.

tions may then rekindle the spark of life; but the body has not within itself the powers of resuscitation, and, if not relieved speedily, dissolution will begin.

Such are some of the wide differences between the operations of the air, and of the food, in sustaining life. Their influence in promoting health, and consequently happiness, both physical and intellectual, and also personal comfort, are equally great and decided. Those who have never observed in their own persons the contrast of the effects of wholesome and unwholesome diet, can not well judge of the value of one over the other, for contrast affords the strongest of all proofs. So those who habitually breathe a tainted and unwholesome air, and especially those whose ignorance prevents them from discerning any impurity in the air, though immediately subject to it, can not appreciate the value of a continued respiration of a well-ventilated atmosphere, in the increased vigor, elasticity, and comfort, of body and mind, which it imparts.

But another, and perhaps a still more important circumstance, is here to be especially noted.

The food which we take into the stomach undergoes, as has been stated, several changes, before it is prepared to enter the circulation. These changes effected, it is finally poured directly into the current of blood, as the latter is about entering the right side of the heart prior to its being transmitted through the lungs. It is not yet blood: it has neither the color, nor the chemical properties, of that important fluid. It has yet to be *sanguified. The air is necessary for this final step.* For this purpose the chyle is brought, in the lungs, in contact with, and is acted upon by, the air in these organs. Without contact with the air, and deriving a vital principle from it, it would still be unfitted to nourish the body. If, therefore, we consider digestion to comprehend *every* step which the food undergoes, from mastication to its conversion into blood, we must consider *respiration as the last act of digestion,* and essential to it. Without the former, the latter function would be useless; for our food, unable to undergo the final change necessary to sustain life, and to replace the worn-out material of the body, would become a burden; without the atmosphere the food would be useless.

One more fact will complete the contrasts of these two sources of animation. Rare are the circumstances, except among the destitute, in which a sufficiency of food can not be obtained; the danger with most persons is on the other hand. Repletion and surfeiting are far more frequent, and productive of great danger. But we can not inhale the air in too great a quantity, or of too pure a quality. The lungs, as well as the stomach, are a digestive apparatus. The one digests *food*, the other *air;* but here the analogy terminates, and one of their principal distinguishing characteristics is, that while the stomach may possibly admit a quantity of food sufficient to paralyze its powers, and even suspend digestion altogether, such is the construction of the lungs, that by their own self-adjusting power, they, under no circumstances, will admit a greater volume of air than is required for the due ventilation of the blood, the sanguification of the food, and for the performance of the other numerous and important processes to which respiration is made subservient.

When pure, air can do no harm, in the greatest amount that it can possibly be inhaled. On the contrary, the greater the amount of food eaten, the greater is the amount of air required to sanguify it; and whether much or little is eaten, the more thoroughly and rapidly it is aerated the better.

With a knowledge of these differences between food

2

and air; of the vast personal, social, and economical benefits derivable from the inhalation of the latter in uniform purity; of its unfailing abundance and facility of attainment; and the ease with which its impurities may be avoided; is it not one of the most surprising facts in the history of civilization, that so much discomfort and ill-health, so premature and so great mortality, as are directly attributable to them, should be permitted?

CHAPTER III.

MECHANISM OF RESPIRATION.

Anatomy of the Chest.—The Ribs.—The Diaphragm.—Action of the Chest—like that of the Bellows —Number of Expansions per Minute. —The Lungs—have no Power of their own to expand.—Internal Structure of the Lungs —Passage of Air in the Lungs audible.—Extent of Surface of Pulmonary Membrane.—Its Object.—Capacity of Lungs for Air—depends on the Muscles of Respiration—and Shape of the Chest. —Exercise important.—Object of Inhalation of Atmospheric Air.—The Heart—a double Organ.—Course of the Blood through it.—Two Circles.—Pulsations of the Heart and Movements of Respiration have Relation to each other.—Number of Pulsations.—Amount of Blood and Air flowing through the Lungs.—Conclusions therefrom.

THE part of the body devoted to the purposes of respiration, is the chest, or thorax. This is composed of the ribs, twelve in number on each side. They have a semicircular shape ; the posterior ends are attached by a moveable joint to the spine behind—and the anterior ends of all but the three lower, made firm by being attached to the breastbone, directly or indirectly, by strips of cartilage. The front ends of the three lower ribs are not attached to any other bone, and are only kept in their places by the muscles, which lie upon, and are attached to, them. The ribs are placed from half an inch to an inch apart, the intermediate spaces being filled by strips of muscle,* passing from one to the other, and which, by their contractions, draw the ribs closer to each other.

* As this term must be used frequently, in the following pages, the reader will understand it to mean that part of the body known as the *lean red flesh ;* its use is to produce motion, and it is the only part of the body which causes motion.

Fig. 1.

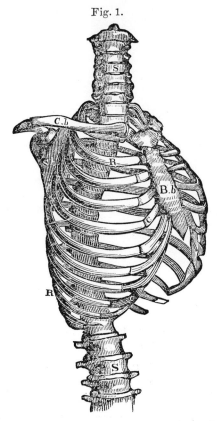

Skeleton of the chest. S, S, the spine. B, b, the breast-bone. R, R, the ribs. C, C, cartilages connecting the ribs with the breast-bone. C, b, the collar bone. S, b, the shoulder-blade. The uppermost ribs are the shortest and most curved, and their lengths increase as they descend.

The chest has, consequently, a conical shape, with its base below, and apex above. The lower boundary or floor of the chest, consists of a very large broad muscle, corresponding in shape to the edge of the base of the cone, and attached to the latter, by its circumference, all around. This muscle, called the *diaphragm*, separates the cavity of the chest from the parts below it, except where a few small apertures allow the bloodvessels, nerves, &c., to pass through to connect with the organs in the abdomen. The diaphragm, in its relaxed state, does not lie flat, but its central portion rises into the thoracic space, so that it presents a deep concavity below, and convexity above. By this arrangement, when the diaphragm contracts, its convexity is reduced, or, in other words, it is partially flattened, whereby the space above it is increased.

Fig. 2.

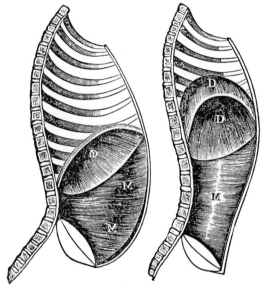

Sections of the chest, diaphragm, and abdomen. D, D, diaphragm. M, M, M, muscles of the abdomen. 1st, the diaphragm in its relaxed condition; 2d, in its contracted state. The difference in the space above it is shown in the two conditions.

On the walls of the chest, externally, are arranged, both behind and in front, several muscles, which, together with the intercostal muscles and diaphragm, form the muscles of respiration. By the contraction of these muscles, the dimensions of the cavity of the chest are increased, in three directions. 1st, by the elevation of the front ends of the ribs, the breastbone is pushed for-

ward, whereby the antero-posterior diameter is length-
ened; 2d, by the same movement, the middle portions
of the ribs are raised and separated farther from each
other, whereby the diameter from side to side is increased; and, 3d, by the depression of the arch of the
diaphragm, which takes place when that muscle is contracted, the vertical diameter is very much increased.
The chest is thus made *to expand* in every direction. By
this expansion, a partial vacuum is created, which can
only be supplied by air through the only opening, *the
mouth*, which is connected with the interior of the chest
by the windpipe. This introduction of air is denominated *inspiration*. Almost immediately after this, *expiration* is produced by the reduction of the various diame-
ters of the chest. This is effected by the action of
certain other muscles, called the antagonist muscles of
respiration. The contained air is thus compressed, and
forced out at the mouth.

These operations are precisely similar in principle to
those of the common bellows. When the two boards
of the bellows are separated, the air rushes in at the
nozzle and valve to fill the vacuum; and when the
boards are pressed together again, the compressed air
is forced out at the nozzle in a powerful stream.

These alternate expansions and contractions of the
chest, amount, on the average, to eighteen a minute.

But the air, strictly speaking, does not enter the chest
itself, but into two large bags, which are always in close
contact with the interior surface of the chest, and are
themselves expanded and diminished in size, as the chest
enlarges and contracts. These large bags are called the
lungs, one of which is placed on each side, having the
heart between them, the three organs occupying nearly
the whole of the thoracic space. The lungs are attached
to the lower end of the windpipe, as it enters the chest

from the neck, and all the air which passes down it, of course, can only get into the lungs.

Fig. 3.

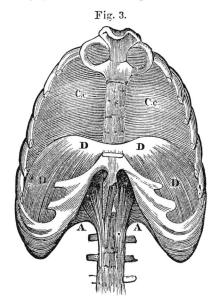

Fig. 3 is a front view of the chest and diaphragm, the latter relaxed. The front half of the ribs being cut away, the interior of the chest is exposed. C, c, C, c, the cavity of the chest, empty. D, D, D, D, the diaphragm, rising high in the centre, and descending very low at the sides and behind. The white space at its upper part is its tendinous portion. A, A, the abdomen.

The nature of this arrangement of the windpipe, lungs, and chest, together with the means by which the diaphragm operates to enlarge the thoracic cavity, are illustrated by a model, of which the following is a figure:—

C, C, fig. 4, is a bell-shaped glass, to represent the chest. In the mouth of the glass is inserted, very tightly, a cork, T, representing the trachea, having a hole lengthwise through it. To the lower end of the cork is attached a small bladder, L, representing a lung. The lower open-

Fig. 4.

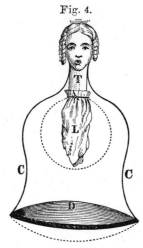

ing of the bell is closed by a piece of sheet gum-elastic, D, which fits air-tight. This answers for the *diaphragm*.

No communication can exist between the cavity of the bell and the external air, except through the hole in the cork; and any air entering through that hole can only go into the bladder. It is evident, also, that when the diaphragm is pushed into the cavity of the glass, as at D, the bladder will be flaccid and void of air; but when the diaphragm is drawn down in the situation of the dotted curve, a partial vacuum in the glass will be the consequence, which can only be supplied with air through the cork, whereby the bladder will expand to its full extent, shown by the dotted circle; and when the diaphragm is pushed up again, the air will be forced out from the bladder.

The diaphragm in the living body does not descend near so low as in the figure; for a very extensive motion is required from it in the latter, to compensate for the want of expansion in the other parts. With this instrument, the model of only one lung can be shown; but it gives us the advantage of *seeing* its mode of action, and the same principle may be applied to both. The

lungs, which are thus the direct recipients of the inhaled
air, correspond exactly, in shape and size, to all those
parts of the cavity of the chest not occupied by the
heart, and a few smaller organs; in expanding and contracting, they follow precisely the movements of the
chest, so that, at all times, they are in contact with its
interior surface.

*But the lungs have no power of their own to expand,
or even to aid in their own expansion.* They are, during
inspiration, entirely passive agents, and follow the motions of the chest without resistance. It is supposed,
however, that they possess a slight degree of *contractil-
ity,* which enables them to contract more readily during
expiration, and thus facilitate the expulsion of the air.
This is as if they were formed of very delicate India-
rubber, which would expand freely on pressure, and
contract slightly when the pressure was removed.

The internal structure of the lungs is very peculiar,
and requires attention at this time. They are not simple
bags, like a bladder, with a free space within, but are
divided and subdivided, to an almost infinite degree, into
very little cells. The whole internal structure of the
lungs is thus a cellular or sponge-like mass, each cell
being so arranged as to connect with the orifice of the
lungs, that it may receive a portion of the air which
enters thereat. The windpipe, at its lower terminus,
is divided into branches, called *bronchiæ,* which pass,
one to each side, and, as they advance, are divided and
subdivided to a great extent, like the branches and twigs
of a tree, terminating finally in the pulmonary cells, in
somewhat the same manner as the twigs terminate in the
leaves of a tree. The lungs appear to the eye to be
composed, almost wholly, of the cells; as the tree, when
in full foliage, appears to be formed almost entirely of
the leaves.

The material of which the lungs and their cells are composed, is *membrane*, of exceeding delicacy, and is translucent. It is so fine as to permit the air to pass through it, yet sufficiently dense to be impervious to the blood.

When the ear is applied to the chest of a healthy person, the sound of the air passing through the bronchiæ and air-cells may be distinctly heard. This has given rise to the invention of the stethoscope, a small wooden trumpet-shaped instrument, which transmits the sounds of respiration, with great distinctness, when one end is placed against the chest, and the other against the ear of the listener. The variations of sound, produced by the modifications of shape in the cells by disease, by the enlargement or contraction of the bronchial tubes, by the presence of various kinds of fluid in them, and other causes, are easily discovered, either through this instrument, or by the naked ear applied to the chest, and are important means of detecting diseases of the pulmonary organs.

From the immense number of the pulmonary air-cells, it will readily be inferred, that the whole surface of the membrane of which they are composed is very great. The air-cells have been estimated to be one hundredth of an inch in diameter, and the extent of surface furnished by them collectively at twenty thousand square inches. By some, the extent of surface they present is supposed to be thirty times that of the external surface of the body.

The purpose of this great extent of surface, is to afford to the air sufficient opportunity to act, readily and speedily, upon the blood, which circulates incessantly through the lungs. The membrane forming the walls of the cells is the means of their communication, as the blood flows through the lungs upon one face of the membrane, while the air is applied to the other, and, by transudation through it, acts upon the fluid.

The blood and air, being by this means divided into a great number of very minute particles, and diffused over this extensive area, act upon each other, in the manner hereafter to be described, most rapidly and effectually.

Many experiments have been tried, for the purpose of ascertaining the capacity of the lungs for air; and the fact has become established, that the lungs *always* contain a large quantity of air. They are never empty. This might be very readily inferred, from the circumstance, already stated, that the external surface of the lungs is in immediate contact, at all times, with the internal surface of the chest. The chest—formed as it is, in a great measure, of unyielding bones, most of them of a semi-circular form—can never have its sides brought into contact with each other, and its cavity, therefore, can not be obliterated, or even reduced to the capacity of its solid contents; and a vacuity must, consequently, always exist, to be filled with air. The amount thus always present in the lungs, varies according to the age, shape of the body, and other circumstances.

The average capacity of the lungs, when the chest is fully expanded, is estimated at twelve pints. At each ordinary expiration, one pint is exhaled, which is replaced by the same amount at each inspiration. There is thus left in the lungs, after an ordinary expiration, eleven pints of air, which keeps the air-cells continually distended.

The greatest inspiration possible, by a strong man, with a well-developed chest, is nine and one fourth pints. Public singers, and those who habitually exercise their lungs to a greater than ordinary degree, by avocations which call for their extra use, especially in the open air, it is ascertained take in from five to seven pints at each inhalation. This enables them to produce a more prolonged expiration, whereby some very interesting effects in vocal and instrumental music can be produced.

The capacity of the chest for inspiration depends, first, upon the strength of the muscles of respiration, and the control the individual may possess over them. These muscles, like nearly all others under the control of the will, are capable of being invigorated and developed by a proper education of them. Well-regulated exercise of any voluntary muscle invariably results in its greater development of size and strength; the quantity of blood transmitted to it is increased by use, and decreased by non-use, increasing its size and power in the former case, and dwindling them away in the latter. This is as true of the respiratory muscles, as of the muscles of the arm or leg. In proportion to their strength, therefore, is their capability of enlarging the chest; and consequently dependent on them, in a considerable degree, is the amount of air which the chest will receive at each inspiration. From this and some preceding remarks, it will be inferred, and very properly, that the popular idea of pain in *the lungs* being produced by hard exercise, and consequent forcible breathing, is erroneous; the pain is not in the lungs, but in the muscles which expand the chest.

The capacity for inspiration, depends, in the second place, upon the shape and position of the chest. If the shoulders are thrown back, the breast-bone put forward, and, especially, if the chest and abdomen are left free from all constraint by clothing or bandages, then the muscles, including the diaphragm, have the most favorable opportunity for action, and the ribs the greatest freedom of motion. But with stooping shoulders, a constrained body, and corseted waist, not only are the ribs prevented from moving freely, but the diaphragm and other muscles, being compressed and uninvigorated, are unable to act with their natural freedom and strength.

Every kind of exercise, and the habits most conducive to an expansion of the thorax and a development of its muscles, should therefore be inculcated. To children, to whom free respiration and abundance of pure air are necessary for their *growth* as well as nourishment, exercise of this part of the body is especially important. Singing, by the regularity with which it brings the respiratory muscles into exercise, and causes a greater development of chest and lungs, is one of the most important exercises to which the young can be trained; and under all the circumstances of life, whether sitting, standing, or lying, asleep or awake, care should be taken by those who have guardianship over them, that no impediment, by position or other circumstances, is in the way of the expansion of their lungs to their fullest extent, and the inhalation of the purest atmosphere.

As already briefly hinted at, one object of the inhalation of atmospheric air, is the purification of the blood. This is proved, not merely by the fact that the blood flows in an incessant current through the lungs, and in immediate proximity to the air-cells, but also by the relative position of the lungs, and the great centre of circulation, the heart. The latter is placed near the centre of the chest, between the two lungs, occupying, with them, nearly the whole of the thoracic cavity. That their anatomical and physiological relations are very intimate, is shown by the number, character, and size of the blood-vessels which pass between them, and the great difference displayed by the blood, before and after it has been transmitted through the lungs, from and to the heart.

The heart is a double organ, having two sides, the right and the left. Each side contains two cavities—

3

a right auricle and ventricle, and a left auricle and ventricle.

The following diagram shows the relative position and mode of communication between these cavities :—

Fig. 5.

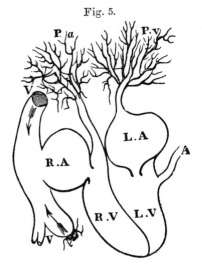

There is no communication between the two sides of the heart, except through the circuit of the lungs, while the chambers of each side are connected with each other, the openings being carefully guarded by valves, which open and shut with every pulsation, admitting the blood through in one direction, but entirely preventing its passage back, like the valves of a pump.

The course taken by the blood is as follows :—

Two large veins (*fig.* 5, V, V)—one descending from the head and upper extremities, the other ascending from the lower extremities, abdomen, and other parts— receive all the impure blood from the body, and unite together near the right auricle (R, A). They pour their joint currents into that chamber, and distend it. When filled, it contracts upon its contents, and forces the fluid into the right ventricle (R, V). This, when filled, con-

tracts, and drives the blood into the pulmonary artery
(P, a), which carries it all to the two lungs, dividing it
between them, through appropriate branches, and dis-
tributing it, in minute particles, over the surface of the
pulmonary air-cells. Its color is yet of a dark purple;
but immediately, as it is distributed through the lungs
and is acted upon by the air in the cells, its color
changes, and becomes a bright vermilion, or scarlet.
This change having been effected, it is again collected
from the lungs by means of another set of blood-vessels,
called pulmonary veins (P, v), which convey it away
from the lungs and carry it back to the heart, where, the
vessels from each lung uniting, it is emptied into the *left*
auricle (L, A). From this it is thrown into the left ventricle (L, V). From this cavity arises the main artery
of the body, the *aorta* (A); and through this great tube
the purified blood is sent, to be distributed all over
the body, visiting every fibre and atom for their sustenance and growth. The final terminations of these dis-
tributing vessels are denominated, from their extreme
minuteness, *capillaries.* These having performed their
office with the red or arterial blood, having deposited the
pure material which they conveyed to the heart, take up
the old and effete matter which requires to be removed,
whereby the blood is changed again to the dark-purple
color which it had before it entered the lungs. In this
impure condition, it is taken up by the capillary *veins,*
and gradually returned to the right side of the heart, at
the point whence we started with this description, to be
again passed through the lungs for purification, and the
restoration of its vermilion color.

The blood thus traverses two circles; — 1st, from the
right side of the heart, through the lungs, to the left side;
and 2d, from the left side, through the body or system,
to the right side of the heart. The first is called the

pulmonary circulation; the second, the *systemic circulation.* In the former, its color is changed from a dark-
purple to a scarlet hue; in the latter, the reverse change
occurs, from the scarlet to the purple.   The first change
is due to the influence of the atmospheric air; the last
change, to the deposite of the pure matter from the
blood, and its taking up the impure to be conveyed out
of the system.

*The pulsations of the heart, and the movements of the
chest in respiration, have a strict relation to each other.*
The purpose of respiration being to introduce into the
lungs the air which is to act upon the blood, sent to the
same organs by the heart, a certain relation as to quantity and frequency must be maintained under all circumstances of health.   Thus in a state of quiescence, when
the heart beats at a certain rate, the number of respirations is exactly proportioned thereto; and when, by
increased exercise of the body, the circulation is stimulated to greater frequency and force, and the blood is
transmitted more rapidly through the lungs, then the
number of respirations is proportionately increased: so
that, under all the varied circumstances of life, there is
found a direct ratio between the frequency of the pulse
and the number of respirations.

*The average number of pulsations of the heart, is
seventy-two per minute.*   In infancy, the number is much
greater, rising to ninety, or even one hundred, per minute.   As age advances, the number is gradually diminished, until, in old age, it will be reduced to sixty, and
sometimes as low as fifty, per minute.

There is, on the average, one respiration to about
every four pulsations of the heart, making the average
number of respirations eighteen per minute.

There are, consequently, in one hour 4,320 pulsations;
and in twenty-four hours the number is 103,680.

The number of respirations in one hour is 1,080 ; and in twenty-four hours, 25,920.

The amount of blood sent to the lungs at each pulsation of the heart, is calculated to be about two ounces. This multiplied by seventy-two (the number of pulsations per minute), gives one hundred and forty-four ounces, or about nine pints of blood sent to the lungs every minute, or sixty-seven and a half gallons per hour.

At each inspiration, forty cubic inches, or about one pint, of air is inhaled : making eighteen pints of air inhaled every minute, or 1,080 pints per hour.

These sums multiplied by twenty-four, respectively, give us the following results :—

Every twenty-four hours, there flow to the lungs sixty hogsheads of air, and thirty hogsheads of blood.

These amounts, apparently so enormous, are the results of accurate and oft-repeated experiments and calculations, and serve well to show the importance, direct and relative, of the influences of the blood and atmosphere upon each other, and upon the condition of the body.

Now, when we consider that it is upon the blood that the body depends for its existence from moment to moment; that to perform its office, the blood must be continually renewed, from a state of impurity (which, if allowed to continue unremoved, will soon prove fatal) to a condition of purity, when it possesses the highest amount of activity; that this change is principally dependent upon the atmosphere taken in at the lungs; the enormous quantities of blood and air which daily pass through the lungs; and that the purer the air inhaled, the better will the blood be fitted to sustain the health and energy of the body;—we have some of the data upon which to base our estimates of the value of fresh and pure air to our health, happiness, and longevity.

3*

CHAPTER IV.

CHEMISTRY OF RESPIRATION.

PART I.—*Effects of Respiration on the Air.*

Atmospheric Air a Compound Gas.—Properties of Nitrogen—Of Oxygen.
—Stimulating Effects of Oxygen.—Carbon in the Blood.—Carbonic
Acid.—Experiments.—Carbonic Acid poisonous—often fatal—Found in
Pits and Wells—Used for Suicidal Purposes.—Aqueous Vapor—Some-
times very copious—How observed.—Damp Air produced by Respira-
tion.—Amount of Water thrown off from the Lungs.

HAVING discussed thus briefly the mechanical relations
of the blood, the air, and the lungs, the next step in the
inquiry refers to the nature of the influence exerted by
respiration on the air and on the blood.

*Atmospheric air is well known to be a compound gas;
its constituents are nitrogen gas and oxygen gas.* Of
these, nitrogen forms four fifths, and oxygen forms one
fifth, of its weight.

These two gases differ greatly in their properties.
Nitrogen, in this connexion, has no decidedly active
properties. It is not a supporter of combustion, nor of
animal life, and yet, *per se*, has no power of destroying
either. If a burning candle, or a small animal, be
immersed in a jar of this gas, the one will cease to burn,
and the other to breathe, but only from the absence of
some supporter of life, or of combustion, and not from
any poisonous or really injurious influence of the nitrogen itself. What its peculiar object, if any, in respiration, or what its action upon the blood, may be, has not

yet been satisfactorily determined. It would seem to be present in the air in such abundance, principally as a diluent of the oxygen, whose properties, in a state of purity, would be too active.

Oxygen, on the other hand, possesses exceedingly powerful properties. It is the presence of this gas in the atmosphere which gives it the power of supporting combustion and animal life, both of which, indeed, consist in, or are maintained by, the combination of oxygen with the carbon of the burning or living body.

When pure, oxygen will cause bodies which are combustible in common air, to burn with greatly-increased rapidity and brilliancy; and many substances which are commonly considered incombustible, will burn readily in this gas.

So animals which breathe at the ordinary rate in common air, have their respiration, circulation, and other animal faculties, stimulated to much more rapid action in pure oxygen.

Of these two components of air, oxygen is, as far as has yet been ascertained, the only sustainer of life. When first discovered, it was, on this account, called *vital air.* It is this which gives to the blood its healthy properties and bright color, and removes from it its impurities. It imparts to the brain, the muscles, the stomach, the heart, and every other organ, a principle which gives them energy and power, and keeps alive the body, by removing from it those substances whose accumulation would soon destroy it.

If the lungs should habitually receive a larger proportion of oxygen than is contained in common air, the operations of the living machine would all be carried on with a degree of animation which would be incompatible with its relations to the other departments of nature, and the animal would soon die from overworking.

The presence of the inert nitrogen, therefore, in such a large proportion, serves the purpose of diluting the stimulating oxygen, and tempering its activity to the degree proper for the just and equable operations of life.

The stimulating effects of inhaling oxygen in a larger proportion than is found in common air, are observable when the nitrous oxyde, or exhilarating gas, is breathed. This prepared gas contains one proportion more of oxygen than is found in the atmosphere, and, when inhaled for a few moments, excites all the animal functions to a much higher degree of energy and force. The muscular system is stimulated to exercise, almost beyond control; the energies of the mind are increased; the circulation is accelerated; and most of the pleasurable functions, such as laughter, speech, &c., are temporarily enhanced. It can only be breathed a few seconds, because of the too great stimulus it affords; and when the containing-vessel is removed from the mouth, and atmospheric air is gradually admitted again to the lungs, these increased effects slowly disappear, and the functions return to their ordinary degree of activity.

This serves to illustrate the influence of oxygen over the animal functions; while, on the other hand, it is easily shown that *a reduction in the amount of this gas, below the quantity found in the purest atmosphere, tends to reduce the energies of the system beneath the standard of health*, giving rise to debilitated bodies, diseases of various organs, general deficiency of strength, or, when carried to too great a degree, to death, more or less sudden.

We will now examine, more particularly, the nature of the changes wrought upon the atmosphere by respiration.

The substance contained in venous or dark blood, which gives it its purple hue, and which is the principal impurity to be removed, is CARBON. This element is better known to us, in a more or less impure form, as charcoal, and, in its purest form, as diamond. Its existence in the dark blood is derived from two principal sources: 1st, from the food; and, 2d, from the various tissues of the body, whose particles are removed to make way for the deposite of pure fresh material from the arterial blood.

From these sources, large quantities of this material, in an extremely subtle form, are constantly added to the blood, and it must of necessity be removed. The oxygen of the air is the agent for its removal. It does it by their being brought into contact, in the lungs, in the manner described. (see chap. 3).

They are thus made to unite with each other chemically, the oxygen, for this purpose, quitting its combination with the nitrogen, and uniting with the carbon, forming a new compound, called *carbonic acid gas.*

As the carbonic acid gas is formed, it is thrown off from the lungs, and discharged into the open air, by expiration.

The nature of the combination which produces carbonic acid in the lungs, is precisely the same as that which produces it when charcoal burns in the open air. In this latter operation, the oxygen is removed from the air and unites with the charcoal, generating carbonic acid gas. These are the only substances whose union will produce that compound; consequently, whenever and wherever it is found, it must have been caused by their combination.

The following experiments will prove that carbonic acid gas is generated in the lungs, and thrown out with the exhaled air : —

Experiment 1*st.* — Take a vial or tumbler full of clear
lime-water; insert in it, to the bottom, a small tube — a
pipe-stem or straw will answer the purpose — and force
the breath through it, so that it will rise through the
liquid in bubbles. In a few minutes the liquid will lose
its transparency, and become of a milky-white color.
This appearance is derived from the presence of carbonate of lime, which floats through the water in a fine,
white, insoluble powder, and which, being heavier, will
soon settle to the bottom when the vessel is at rest, and
may then be separated by decanting off the liquor.

Experiment 2*d.* — When the powder has been separated and partly dried, if a few drops of muriatic acid,
or spirit-of-salt, are added to it, it will be decomposed,
and a gas will be disengaged from it, with considerable
effervescence, which, if collected in a receiver, may be
proved to be carbonic acid gas.

In this manner the formation of carbonate of lime is
proved, the carbonic acid of which could only have been
derived from the expired breath, proving to us that carbon is taken from the blood in the lungs, by means of
the oxygen of the air, and both are returned to the air
in the form of the compound gas.

Further experiments, which need not here be detailed
(those described may be tried by any one), have clearly
demonstrated that the quantity of oxygen which is lost
by the air, is precisely the amount necessary to account
for the carbonic acid which is thrown off from the lungs.

The nitrogen gas, which forms so large a proportion
of the air, and which, of course, is inhaled with the
oxygen, is returned to the air in very nearly, or quite the
same amount as it is taken in, the only difference being
its separation from the oxygen   Little or none (experiments vary somewhat on this point) appears to be lost
by the process of respiration.

Two important facts are, therefore, proved by the experiments which have been instituted for ascertaining the changes produced by respiration: 1st, that oxygen gas, the only vivifying principle of the atmosphere, loses its elementary freedom; and, 2d, its place is supplied by another and a compound gas, carbonic acid. This latter, we will now proceed to show, is directly the opposite of oxygen, as regards the support of life and combustion: —

Experiment 3d.—In the bottom of a quart or pint jar, place a tablespoonful of pulverized marble; pour on it a few drops of muriatic acid. Immediately an effervescence of gas will take place: this gas is carbonic acid, and is identical in character with that exhaled from the lungs, except being purer. Its weight being greater than that of common air, as it is freed from the marble, it remains, and expels the common air from the jar. When the jar is full, if a lighted candle is immersed in it, it will be instantly extinguished, as if dipped in water; or if a mouse or other small animal be put into it, death will ensue, sooner than if immersed in water.

These results demonstrate not only the inability of carbonic acid gas to support life and combustion, but, in the case of the small animal, there is indicated a positive activity for the destruction of life. It is thus proved to us that this gas is *poisonous.* When an animal is immersed in water, or in nitrogen gas, its death is not instantaneous, because they are not, *per se,* destructive of life —the animal dies merely for want of oxygen to decarbonize the blood; and several minutes, or even an hour or two, may elapse ere the undecarbonized blood will have exerted its full influence upon the brain and other organs, to destroy the vital spark. But when pure carbonic acid is inhaled, it exerts a specific influence, of an exceedingly poisonous character, which causes an almost immediate destruction of vitality after its first inhalation. It is said of the Grotto-del-Cane, in Italy,— the floor of which is covered, to the depth of several inches, with this gas from a natural source — that when dogs are taken into it, they immediately sink down, apparently lifeless, but are restored by being dragged into the open air. This may seem to oppose the view just presented of the deadly-poisonous nature of the gas; but, upon examination, it will not appear to. The gas emanating from the soil can not be supposed entirely pure, and must, as the mouth of the cave is open, be more or less combined with atmospheric air. Its destructive agency is, therefore, only partially exerted.

In long-closed wells and pits, this gas will sometimes accumulate to a considerable depth, destroying the lives of those who enter them. Its presence may be instantly detected by lowering a lighted candle into the well. Fatal effects have frequently ensued from breathing carbonic acid gas from burning charcoal in close rooms. It is said to have been employed for suicidal purposes; and the sensations produced by it, as by its increasing volume it gradually overcomes the faculties, are said to be rather pleasurable than otherwise.

Closely connected with this subject, is that of the aqueous vapor contained in the air expired. Some have assumed this to be a direct product of respiration depending on a supposed excess of oxygen combining with the hydrogen of the blood; while others say it is a mere secretion from the membrane lining the pulmonary passages. This difference of opinion, however, does not affect, in any degree, the important conclusion that large quantities of it are exhaled continually. This is apparent to all in cold weather, from the cloud which issues from the mouth at each expiration; or by breathing on a cold stone or glass, when it will condense in such quantities as to form in drops. Players on wind instruments often find the notes obstructed by the copious collections of the fluid, condensed from the breath, in the tubes of their instruments. This is poured out from the lungs at all times—not only in winter, when it is so apparent to the eye, but also in summer, or in a warm room, when it is imperceptible under ordinary circumstances. Most persons must have noticed the abundant dew-like collections of water upon the inside of the windows of a church, or other room, when occupied by many people in a cold day,—giving a clear indication of the vapory condition of the whole atmosphere within; for it is only from that part of the atmosphere immediately adjacent to, and in contact with the glass, that the vapor is condensed.

In consequence of the concentration of so great an amount of vapor, all the attributes and influences of a "damp air," so generally and justly believed injurious to health, are exerted within the room, though the external atmosphere may be clear and dry.

The amount of vapor discharged from the lungs, varies with circumstances within and without the body; thus the hygrometric state of the atmosphere exerts a considerable influence over the quantity discharged; for if the atmosphere is surcharged with moisture already, according to the laws of evaporation, the surface of the lungs can not emit the same quantity as when the atmosphere is dry, and more capable of absorbing the vapor.

The retention of this aqueous vapor in damp weather will account, in some degree, for the feelings of oppression experienced by most persons in that condition of the atmosphere, and the greater elasticity and vigor enjoyed in dry weather, especially when accompanied by brisk winds from the north or northwest.

4

In the same manner does the atmosphere of a crowded room operate to prevent the exhalation of vapor, and produce the oppressed feelings incident to a damp air; and this, though the external air may be dry and clear.

From various experiments upon this subject, the average amount of watery vapor exhaled from the pulmonary air-cells, has been determined to be about twenty ounces, or nearly a pint and a quarter of liquid in twenty-four hours.

Carbon and watery vapor are therefore the two substances, which it is the office of the lungs to remove from the blood, — whose retention serves, though in very different degrees, to impair its purity, and to render it unfit to perform its important duties healthfully. To reinhale the carbonic acid gas, which we have seen is a poisonous material, or to prevent the free escape of the vapor, is with the latter to burden the system with an oppressive substance, and with the former to endanger its soundness, and to lay the foundation of disease.

A means of free escape from the immediate precincts of the body, and from any liability of re-inhalation of these two substances, is second only, if at all, in importance, to a plentiful supply of fresh, pure, dry air, for respiration.

CHAPTER V.

CHEMISTRY OF RESPIRATION.

PART II.—*Effect of Respiration on the Blood.*

Questions to be considered.—Difference between Venous and Arterial
Blood.—Intimate Relation between the Circulation and Respiration.—
Panting.—Influence of Respiration on the Flow of Blood.—Illustrations.
—Why is Carbon found in the Blood?—Its Source—Temperature of
the Body—How maintained—Same in all Climates.—The Skin its
Regulator.—The Safety-Valve.—Fever.—Influence of the Skin upon it.

FROM the foregoing description of the changes
wrought upon the air, we next pass to consider—

*The nature of the changes which Respiration exerts
upon the blood.* Three questions here arise for consideration: 1st, What are the condition and appearance of
the blood when flowing into the lungs?—2d, What are
its appearance and condition when flowing from the
lungs?—and, 3d, What has produced the change?

The anatomical relations of the heart and lungs have
been pointed out. The right side of the heart receives
all the blood from the body, preparatory to its being
sent to the lungs; the left side of the heart receives it
from the lungs, preparatory to its being distributed again
through the body. In the right side of the heart, the
blood possesses a very dark modena, or purple hue,
sometimes nearly black,—and, being brought by the
veins, and having almost uniformly the same appearance
in that set of vessels throughout, it is called *venous
blood.*

In this condition it goes into the lungs, where it is brought in contact with the respired air; and immediately as it is acted upon by the air, its color is changed to a bright vermilion, or scarlet. This change of color would alone be indicative of some important alteration of its chemical constitution; but, in addition to this, we have, as already stated, a conclusive proof of the removal of carbon, by the presence of this element in the air which is exhaled.

If further evidence is wanted, that these changes in the color and chemical property of the blood are due to the atmosphere, it is found in experiments made to test the action of air on blood out of the body, which may easily be repeated. Thus, if a clot of venous blood be introduced into a close vessel containing air, the clot speedily passes from a purple to a scarlet color; and if the air contained in the vessel be analyzed, it is found that a portion of its oxygen has disappeared, and been replaced by a proportionate quantity of carbonic acid. If the clot be exposed to pure oxygen, this change takes place more rapidly, and to a greater extent; if the air contain no oxygen, no change of color takes place. The direct and immediate effect of the air upon the blood, is, therefore, to free it from a quantity of carbon and hydrogen; the first to form carbonic acid,—the second, watery vapor, with the oxygen of the air.

These circumstances demonstrate an intimate relation between the circulation and respiration. This is, indeed, made manifest in ordinary, by the increased action of *both*, when one or the other is stimulated to unusual action. Thus, when the body is subjected to extra exertion, as in running or laboring, the circulation is more or less accelerated, and, in a proportional degree, the respiration is increased in frequency; so that the blood, which is thus driven with greater rapidity through

the lungs as well as through the body, may be supplied
with oxygen in proportion to the increased demand.   In
a state of repose, the number of respirations is, to the
number of pulsations of the heart, as one to four —
eighteen to seventy-two in the minute.   When the body
is in active exercise, the number of pulsations is increased to eighty, or even ninety, per minute ; and then,
also, the respirations increase in number, *pari passu.*
And not only this, but the expansion of the chest is
also augmented.   This produces the *panting* of the
horse, or the dog, after a hard run.   In some diseases,
also, as in fever, the same relative action is maintained ;
the pulse is generally accelerated, sometimes to the
extent of one hundred and fifty per minute, and the
number of respirations in proportion.   In infancy, man-
hood, and old age, the pulse varies ; frequent in the first,
at a medium in the second, and few in the last period ;
the number of respiratory movements takes the same
variation, maintaining the same relative proportion
throughout.

But the intimacy of this relation is closer than is
generally understood, even by some who may be more
than ordinarily conversant with the operations of animal
physiology.   For a minute knowledge of this, we are
indebted to the observations of modern science.   Nearly
every point of interest in the circulation of the blood
through the body, was established soon after the discovery of the circulation by Harvey, in the early part
of the seventeenth century; but it is only within a comparatively recent period that the pulmonary circulation,
and the important relation which it bears to the movements of the chest, and the chemical relations of the air
and blood, have become understood.

It is established by direct experiment, that the movements of the chest in expiration and inspiration have a

4*

bearing upon the flow of blood to, and its discharge
from, the lungs.

Thus, at the instant that the lung is receiving a fresh
supply of air in inspiration, its expansion gives an occasion for an increased flow of blood also, forced in by
the contraction of the right ventricle of the heart.   And
it is evident, that, during the expansion of the lungs, an
elongation of the branches of the pulmonary artery will
take place, and into this vacuum the blood will be
absorbed, independent of its projectile force from the
heart itself.   A current of air and a stream of blood are
thus simultaneously received by the lungs.

By expiration, on the other hand, the lung is partially
collapsed, and its bulk diminished; the compression of
the air-vesicles, which expels the air, acts also on the
blood, now converted into arterial, and assists its pro-
pulsion to the left side of the heart, to be thence transmitted through the body.   There is, therefore, a relation
existing between the movement of the chest in expiration and the action of the left side of the heart, and in
inspiration with the right side of the heart.

"If the great vessel which returns the blood to the
heart, called the jugular vein, be exposed to view in a
living animal, it is seen to be alternately filled and
emptied, according to the different states of inspiration
and expiration.   It becomes nearly empty at the moment
of inspiration; because, at that moment, the venous
stream is hurried forward to the right chambers of the
heart, which, in consequence of the general dilation of
the chest, are now expanded to receive it.   This may
be rendered still more strikingly manifest to the eye: if
a glass tube, blown at the middle into a globular form,
be inserted by its extremities into the jugular vein of a
living animal, in such a manner that the venous stream
must pass through this globe, it is found that this globe

becomes nearly empty during inspiration, and nearly full during expiration; — empty during inspiration because, during this action, the blood flows forward to the right chambers of the heart; full during expiration because, during this action, the venous stream being retarded in its passage through the lung, its motion becomes so slow in the jugular vein, there is time for its accumulation in the glass globe."* In the carotid artery, on the contrary, which carries the blood to the head, and runs near the jugular vein, the opposite result takes place.

It is stated by Dr. Southwood Smith, that in the course of some experiments performed by Dr. Dill and himself, for the purpose of ascertaining more precisely the relation between the circulation and respiration, a phenomenon was observed, which places these points in a still more striking and clear light. The jugular vein happened to be divided. The vessel ceased to bleed during inspiration; but as soon as expiration commenced, began to bleed copiously; which is the reverse of what uniformly happens in the entire state of the vessel. The reason for this, as explained by Dr. Smith, is, that the division of the vein cuts off its communication with the lung, removes it from the influence of respiration, brings it under the sole influence of the arterial current, and consequently reverses its natural condition, and so reverses the manner in which its current flows; affording a beautiful illustration of the influence of the two actions of respiration on the two sets of blood-vessels concerned in the function.

The facts of the presence of carbon in the blood, and of the necessity for its removal therefrom, are demonstrated beyond all cavil.

But when it is regarded as an impurity, and the purification of the blood from its presence is proved neces-

* Philosophy of Health, vol. ii., p. 71.

sary for the maintenance of the life and health of the body, there arise several very interesting physiological inquiries ; — why, as it must be removed, is it found in so great quantity ? whence its source ? and what useful purpose is gained by its existence there ?

These points, though not at first sight possessing any important relation to our immediate subject, " the importance of pure air," will be found, on due investigation, to be very intimately concerned with it, and necessary to be understood, in order to a full and clear appreciation of the general topic.

The principal source of the carbon of the blood, as already stated, is the food.

All vegetable and animal substances are well known to be constituted, in large part, of this element. By the digestive process, the food is so acted upon, that the relations of its component elements are greatly changed, and they are rendered capable of readily forming new combinations with other elements with which they may be brought in contact. Thus the carbon of the food, which before the digestive process, exhibits very little tendency to unite with the oxygen of the air, and none at all without its original relations being altered, is so disengaged from its combinations by digestion, as to enable it to quit its union with the other elements of the food, and unite with the oxygen of the air in the lungs, at the moment of contact with it.

The great object of the presence of so much carbon in the blood, and of its removal therefrom, by the function of respiration, is undoubtedly the *maintenance of the warmth of the body.* It has been already remarked, that the combination of carbon and oxygen in the lungs, is a process precisely similar in effect, to a union of the same substances out of the body ; — the result in the latter case is the evolution of caloric, made apparent to the sense; it is the same in the lungs, whence the heat is distributed over the body, by means of the circulating blood. Carbonic acid, also, is evolved in both instances.

The power possessed by animals, of sustaining a temperature above that ordinarily found in surrounding objects, and the uniformity of their temperature (ninety-eight degrees, Fahrenheit), in even the coldest latitudes, as well as in the torrid zone, where the external temperature is often much higher, are remarkable phenomena. The sustained temperature of the living body, under a concurrence of circumstances, tending constantly to depress it, is solely due to the evolution of caloric by the chemical admixture of carbon and oxygen, brought in contact with each other by the process of respiration. This is admitted by all physiologists who have investigated the subject, though there is a difference of opinion as to the exact point where the union is made, some maintaining that the oxygen is absorbed by the blood as it flows through the lungs, and that it unites with the carbon at the more distant points of the arterial circulation, as, particle by particle, it is brought into proximity with it; and that the heat is thus developed where it is most needed, viz., in the capillary circulation and on the surface of the body. By others it is believed that the union of the two is effected in the lungs, and that the heat, which would then be supposed to be greatest at this point, is not allowed to accumulate there, by the rapidity of the circulation removing it as fast as generated.

In a work of this kind, it would be neither necessary nor appropriate to occupy space, by the presentation of the arguments on either side of this question, conceding, as they both do, the main fact, that *the temperature of the body is due to the combustion of its carbon.* The difference is only as to the place where this combustion occurs. The necessity of oxygen for this purpose, as well as for the purification of the blood, is therefore indisputable,—and equally clear is the necessity for having the oxygen in the greatest possible purity and abundance in the atmosphere.

The fact of the temperature of the body being the same in all climates, has already been adverted to. At first view it may seem somewhat surprising, that, in the frigid regions of Labrador and Greenland, where the external temperature is often more than one hundred degrees lower than that of the body, there should be an equal facility for sustaining it, as in the land of the Amazon and Malay, where the temperature of the air and body are nearly alike. This surprise will in some measure abate upon the recollection of the superior facilities presented in the north for retaining the warmth of the body, by clothing of furs, &c. ;—it is still further lessened on calling to mind the colder and more condensed atmosphere, and the consequently greater amount of oxygen inhaled in the same bulk of air ; it is removed, when the nature of the food of the inhabitants of those regions is considered, being composed, in great part, of fatty and oily substances, which contain a larger proportion of carbon, by which the blood is supplied with this element to an amount proportionate to the oxygen inhaled. The combustion of this larger amount of carbon, of course develops a proportionately large amount of caloric, to compensate for its greater abstraction by the external cold.

In the higher latitudes, there is a continual tendency to a depressed temperature, requiring the consumption of an extraordinary amount of oxygen, and a more rapid development of heat; in the equatorial regions, on the other hand, the tendency is rather the other way, as is the case, also, in the temperate regions during the heats of summer. Some means is there required to keep down the temperature of the body—to prevent the oppression and excitement incident to these different circumstances. A compensating power is found in the external surface of the body: the skin is the great *regulator* of the temperature. The perspiration which it exhales, in quantities greater or less according to the external heat, or the activity of the circulation, evaporates, and, by this evaporation, carries off the surplus caloric, till the temperature of the body is reduced to its proper standard. Every one is aware, that in the winter season, the fluid of perspiration is much less in amount where the external air is much colder than the body; and is very copious in the summer, where the operations of the living body tend to the production of more caloric than would be comfortable or salubrious; the skin, by its perspiration, acts in both extremes, and at every intermediate point, as a *safety-valve*, opening its pores to let off the accumulating caloric in the one case, and closing them to prevent its escape in the other. The most delicate sympathy is thus exercised between the generator and regulator of animal caloric.

There is a condition of the system, frequently occurring, in which the great value of this regulator is evinced by the non-performance of its function. In the disease called *fever*, the circulation and respiration are carried on with unnatural activity, and there is, consequently, a superabundant amount of caloric developed; the action of the skin being checked at the same time, it remains dry, there is no perspiration to remove the surplus heat, and the whole system, consequently, feels the injurious and oppressive effect of its accumulation. It is then one of the first objects of the physician to restore the function of the skin, to reinduce the perspiration, and in this way to diminish the disease, and relieve the sufferer.

CHAPTER VI.

Different Circumstances of Human Life noticed.—The Infant.—The Scholar.—The Apprentice.—Out-Door and In-Door Labor contrasted.— Workshops.— The Journeyman.— The Sailor.— The Printer.— The Farmer.— Shoemakers and Tailors.—Crowds in the Open Air.— Amount of Vitiation of Air proportioned to the Number of People and Length of Time.—Anecdote.— Dormitories.—Hotels.—Steamboats.— The "Oregon."—Rail-Cars.—Omnibuses.

LET us follow the human being through the various periods and circumstances of his life, and observe with what degree of freedom the atmosphere is allowed to exert the full influence of its invigorating powers upon him.

First—*as the tender Infant*—he scarcely has made his entrance into the great ocean of air, and uttered his plaintive petition for a portion of the new element to expand his little chest, ere, by the careful nurse, he is tucked away under the coverlid, with his head closely wrapped in a blanket-shawl, lest the already impure air of the chamber should be too strong for his weak organs.

Should an anxious aunt, led by her curiosity, throw off a fold of the mummy-like case,—or should the infant in its suffocative throes, penetrate an opening through the woollen walls which confine it, his little throat, expand-ing instinctively with the touch of a somewhat better air, greets it with swelling notes of mournful joy. Alas! it is but the signal for the good nurse to "*protect*" the babe against the danger of *taking cold,* in an atmosphere of perhaps ninety degrees Fahrenheit. She has no notion that her delicate charge shall get the sniffles by undue and premature exposure. The louder little Oliver cries for more oxygen, the closer is he confined to hush his noise.

His next position is as the *Schoolboy;* — and here we find him, with from five to five hundred others, immured between close walls,—perhaps in a low-ceiled apartment, half under ground,—with doors and windows closed, and calked tight, to save the heat from the fuel burning in a little red-hot stove, and exhausting a large portion of what little oxygen there may be present in the air. His brain is stimulated by threats of punishment or hopes of reward; his body is constrained within the narrowest limits; motion is denied him; and his tender and growing muscles are forbidden to participate, as they should, in even the poor nourishment which the imperfectly oxygenized blood might furnish. At night he occupies a room, rather larger than a prison-cell, which contains sufficient air to allow him to breathe it in its purity for the space of from thirty to sixty minutes; after which, as the room is so small, for fear the night-air will blow right on him, if the window-sash should be lowered to give an exit to some of the foul air, he inhales and re-inhales, in larger and larger proportion, the carbonic acid thrown off from his own lungs as excrementitious poison, until, in the morning, he creeps from his bed in a dripping sweat, drooping, languid, and unrefreshed by his sleep, and poorly fitted to engage in the severe mental task imposed upon him by his teacher.

Can we wonder that he should "creep like snail, unwillingly to school," where the artificial stimulus of the rod, is substituted for the natural stimulus of oxygen?

The next period of his life is as *the Apprentice.* In very few of the various trades, or professions, is he sub-

5

jected, during the hours of labor, to any other atmosphere than such as is polluted, by either the respiration
of numbers of persons in a small room, or the effluvia
of materials of manufacture, increased and concentrated
by the back situation and narrow enclosure of the house
itself, by which all visitation of genial atmospheric currents is prevented.

There are some trades, which, happily for their followers, require the labor to be performed in the open
air; such are those of the house-builder, the ship-builder,
farmer, gardener, and some others; but the laborers at
these occupations, at night are generally subject to
vitiated air, in small crowded chambers, whereby the
good effects of the exposure of the day are greatly
counteracted. But all others, at least those pursuing
mechanical trades, pass their working hours in close,
unventilated shops, redolent with the fumes of steam,
smoke, white-lead, sour paste, acids, alkalies, the gases
from decomposing animal and vegetable matters, and
many other matters, which add more or less to the deleterious properties of the air respired by many lungs.

A ventilated workshop is almost an unknown thing;
and he who decides upon himself, or his child, becoming
an apprentice to any one of the great majority of trades,
must calculate upon a prostration of strength, paleness
of countenance, languor of spirits and body, frequent
sickness, and almost inevitably, as statistics show, a
premature death.

This results, too, in very many of these occupations,
without the action of any peculiar cause connected with
them. A large proportion of the evil is believed to be
due to the foulness of the atmosphere necessarily produced by the absence of ventilation.

Yet those avocations in which the presence of deleterious gases is unavoidable, may be almost, if not entirely,

disarmed of their evil influences, by a proper system of ventilation, which would conduct the effluvia away from the operatives, to be dispersed in the open air.

Should the apprentice survive these continued aggressions upon his vital energies, and arrive at the years of *journeymanship*, he is not likely to bring to the aid of his employer a thoroughly-invigorated body, and consequently is, more or less, deficient in the strength and skill which constitute his capital in business. The foundation upon which his life has been laid, is, as it were, softened; and the circumstances in which he lives and labors are no better calculated to improve and strengthen it.

The value of the strength, talent, and skill, which are thus lost, to both masters and workmen, is incalculable, as are the privations and sufferings to individuals, families, and states, produced by an entire neglect of this most important means of preserving health and life.

The laborer who, in the exercise of his vocation, enjoys the atmosphere in its greatest purity, is the *Sailor*. On the ocean, away from the effluvia and gases generated on land, with nothing near him that can produce more than a momentary injury, he inhales the pure air, on deck or aloft, in most copious draughts, and at moments, when muscular exercise and mental energy are at their utmost, and all the elements of life and strength conspire to render him healthful and vigorous. But when relieved from duty, where do we find him ? — down in the forecastle, a close and narrow place, reached by a single small entrance, usually shut tight to exclude the light and noise, that he may take his rest, with a dozen or more others, inhaling an atmosphere as impure as that above is pure. The healthful circumstances of his life " on deck" are thus counteracted and overcome, by the few hours during which he is "turned in," to seek the benefit of balmy sleep.

Jack rarely lives to a ripe old age. This fact is doubtless attributable, in some degree, to his proverbially dissipated life, to the hardships he endures at sea, and to the absence of those comforts more generally enjoyed by landsmen.

But it must not be overlooked, that in the active pursuit of his avocation, the circumstances legitimately connected with it are pre-eminently disposed to invigorate him ; and that their value is destroyed, and their good influences annulled, by his confinement with numbers of others in a small, crowded, dirty, and totally unventilated apartment, — for which latter adjective there can be no valid excuse.

The same remarks apply, with nearly equal force, to the *Farmer*, whose occupation and general habits of life are most of all conducive to health and longevity. His exposure to free air — his regular and unexciting labor, never exhausting him as does the sailor's — his protection from storms — the smooth and even tenor of his ways, — are altogether provocative of the most exuberant health and happinesss. He subjects himself to but one drawback, — his nights are too often passed in an area too small to supply him with unadulterated air during all his sleeping hours. The house of the countryman is almost proverbially small, the chambers low-ceiled, and ventilation never thought of. Thus, the happy effects of his position by day are, in a great measure, counteracted by that of the night; and, as will be shown in subsequent chapters, the seeds of disease may be sown during the brief hours of sleep, which the purer and healthier circumstances of the day may never eradicate.

Probably no operatives suffer more from the inhalation of air rendered impure by respiration, than *Printers*, —particularly that branch of the craft called compositors. Especially is this the case with those who work on the morning newspapers; as any one who will pay a visit to the composing-room at midnight, in cold weather, will readily believe. The uppermost room in the building is generally occupied for this purpose, and, like all upper stories, has a low ceiling. That the workmen may finger the types with facility and rapidity, the metal, as well as the hands, must be at a comfortable temperature. This requires a high temperature of room, generally raised by stoves. That he may read the manuscript, a strong light is produced by some powerful burner near his head. Standing still for hours, no muscular exercise gives activity to his circulation; while from long-continued breathing of an air whose vital property is rapidly destroyed by combustion of fuel and oil, the respiration of many individuals, and the expansive power of the heat, we find his countenance pale, his muscles small and flabby, his chest narrow, his nervous system too sensitive to permit the smallest current of fresh air to touch him, his appetite and digestion feeble, presenting a *tout ensemble* of condition, the sure precursor of an early grave. Who sees an aged printer, still standing at the case ?

Subject to difficulties of a similar character, in some respects rather better, in others worse, are two other classes of operatives—*Shoemakers and Tailors.* The hot, close, and small rooms, the sitting and cramped postures, the deficient exercise, the unintellectual character of the occupations, combined with the universal absence of ventilation, render these avocations as fatal to health and life as any in which the laborer is not directly exposed to noxious fumes.

It would be needless to multiply instances of trades in

5*

which, from the rejection of the means whence might be derived a much greater amount of comfort, health, energy, and years, there is an incalculable loss of all these, not only to the laborers themselves, and their families, but, in addition, to the employers, of time, talent, and money. Resting upon the broad and indisputable fact, that pure air is the great supporter of life, and health, not only of the body, but of the intellect, it must be conceded in reason, as it is established in proof, that mankind does, both in the relation of employer and employee, suffer a privation, more or less great, of all the benefits, moral, physical, and pecuniary, that naturally flow from a sound and healthy condition of mind and body.

In pursuing this elucidation, we find the evil is not confined to the laboring classes, or to the less intelligent portions of society. Wherever we find a civilized being domiciled, whether pursuing interest, pleasure, worship, or justice, alone or in society, at home or travelling, we find him breathing an atmosphere more or less impure. Very often the effects are demonstrated at the moment, in flushings of face, perspiration, drowsiness, headaches, vertigo, and fainting, and very frequently at more remote periods, by the developments of more profound and serious diseases of the lungs, heart, head, or stomach.

For the immediate effects, we need but look into almost any court-room, church, lecture-room, theatre, ball-room, or place of assembly of any name, where many persons are crowded together without ventilation, and that is in almost *every one* yet known. Nay, one need but form one of a numerous crowd in the *open air*, in a day when the atmosphere is perfectly still, to feel the oppressive effects of an insufficiency of pure air.

This has been the experience of many a one, in the crowded meetings which assemble occasionally on the

platform in the Park, in front of the City-Hall, a spot
very advantageous for both speakers and hearers, but
whose sheltered position on certain days, renders the air
decidedly oppressive, though it has neither walls nor
roof to confine it.

The volume of carbonic acid gas and watery vapor
which are exhaled from the lungs of the crowd, together
with the other natural corporeal emanations, accumulate
to so great a degree under such circumstances, as to require a long time to escape, when there is no current of
air to disperse them; and it is not an unknown thing for
some to fall faint and exhausted under the want of air,
even with the canopy of heaven in full view, and its deep
ocean of air, within a few feet, in perfect purity.

If such things come to pass in the *open air*, where
these accumulations would, *a priori*, be supposed impossible, how much worse must it it be with a crowd confined within impervious walls and roof, having the air
artificially heated, and lighted by the glare of burning
gas or oil, both of which aid powerfully in using up the
oxygen, while there is no means for a due supply of it
from without.

The foolishness of human wisdom can scarce go
further.

There is indeed scarcely a position in which a civilized
being can be placed, in which he is not subjected, in a
greater or less degree, to a vitiated atmosphere. It is
not only in the public assembly, or the private soiree, the
church, or the court-room, that he breathes an air which
has already been inhaled by his own or others' lungs; —
but it is also in his private chamber, in his parlor, kitchen,
office, store, or workshop, that we find him confined
to an atmosphere incapable of ready renewal. The
fact that he erects a house with solid walls, and covers
it with an impervious roof, thus separating for his own

exclusive use, a small portion of the great atmospheric ocean, in which he immures himself, and exerts his ingenuity to exclude any more of the vital fluid :—this fact alone is evidence of the unnaturalness of his position and habits, and of his ignorance or disregard of one great duty to himself and family.

The air breathed by a single individual becomes deoxygenized in proportion to that breathed by a score or a hundred—and in a proportionate length of time a quantity of unventilated air will become as thoroughly foul and unwholesome, under the operation of a single pair of lungs, as of any greater number. The number of people, and the amount of air, are relative merely :— vitiation of the latter, and danger to the former, are alike inevitable and avoidable.

So universal is inattention to supplies of fresh air in private dwellings, even the most palaceous, it were almost a work of supererogation to quote an instance of the effects of the impure air upon their inmates, but one case which came to the writer's personal notice, was so striking, as to be deemed worthy of record.

In the month of December, 184–, in the evening of a day remarkable for the intense coldness of the air, the thermometer being twelve degrees below freezing, the executive committee of an important charitable institution assembled in the house of one of its members, a professional gentlemen, residing at the corner of two of the most fashionable streets. Twenty-one were present, and occupied an apartment about eighteen feet square. The principal hall of the house was warmed by a large Nott's stove, and in the room occupied by the committee an additional stove was necessary to make it comfortable. The builder of the house had evidently performed his duty faithfully, for the doors and windows fitted their frames with accuracy, preventing as much as possible any ingress of air from without, or any exit of that within.

Here were assembled judges, physicians, merchants, editors, and others, of the highest standing for intelligence and philanthropy. For a short time the business went on, under the direction of the able chairman, with despatch. Soon he began to complain of the closeness of the room, and opened the door leading to the hall, and placed himself in the opening. He was cautioned against " catching cold," but his feelings of oppression overruled all such scruples. Unsatisfied with the air from the hall, scarcely better than that of the room, he went to a window on the opposite side, and, lowering the upper sash some six inches, placed himself directly under it, to allow the cold external air to fall immediately upon his feverish head. This movement was a signal for a general disruption of the committee, and the effects of the atmosphere upon the different individuals in the room, was watched with no little interest by those who knew too well the true cause of the difficulty.

The cases of three of the gentlemen will be offered as examples of the varied effect of deficient or impure air upon different constitutions and temperaments. They sat upon the same sofa. One was a gentleman alike venerable for his years and lore, one of the most active members of the institution ; another was in the prime of life, enjoying a high reputation as a lawyer, and of distinguished name in the ranks of literature ; between them was seated a universally respected professor in a medical school, who has since been carried to the grave.

The first-mentioned complained of the *great heat* of the room, and wished the fire might be extinguished ; the second said he felt *very cold*, even in that high temperature, and actually rose and *put on his greatcoat;*

while the third, as if mysteriously influenced by the two
extremes by which he was flanked, complained of alternate feverishness and chilliness, and expressed himself
unable to account for the singular sensations.

Thus was given an exhibition of the manner in which
different temperaments are affected by one cause, which
in this case was undoubtedly a deficiency of oxygen gas
in the atmosphere, that important principle having been
in a great measure consumed by the respiration of the
company, the burning of the fuel in the stove, and of the
gas and candles, while the high temperature served to
rarify the air, and thus reduce the quantity below what
it would otherwise have been. Doubtless a good system
of ventilation would have obviated the whole difficulty,
and avoided evils for which neither the beautiful paint-
ings, the costly furniture, nor the downy carpets, could
compensate.

Of the various apartments of the wealthier, as well as
the poorer, class of dwellings, the worst for health, in
respect to the atmosphere, are doubtless the *dormitories.*
The reasons for this distinction are obvious: 1st, they
are occupied for a greater number of successive hours.
2d, during the hours of sleep, there are no opening and
shutting of doors and windows, no movements of persons or furniture, which, in rooms occupied in the daytime, produce more or less motion, and consequently
change, in the air. 3d, fires, which always cause currents in the air, are, during the hours of sleep, extinguished, and the doors and windows of the apartment
are generally shut close, from apprehension of the effects
of night-air. 4th, from the quiescent state of the atmosphere of bed-rooms, the poisonous emanations from the
body move off, and become mingled with the adjacent
air more slowly, and hence are more readily reinhaled.
5th, the relative dimensions of parlors and chambers are

almost universally, as the previous reasoning will show, inversely what they should be. The longer occupation of a bed-room at night, without any means of a renewal of the air, requires a proportionate larger amount of it for healthful respiration : whereas we find the bed-room actually of smaller dimensions.

There are few persons who have not noticed the peculiar disagreeable odor of a bed-room in the morning, after a night's occupation by only two persons. If any reader should happen not to have noticed it, let him leave his chamber, some morning, and after spending half an hour in the open air, return to it. If it has been undisturbed during his absence, his senses will at once discover the condition of the contained air, and he will be able to appreciate the nauseous nature of the gases he has been inhaling for hours. He may then be able to account for his unrefreshed feelings, and no longer wonder that he should rise in the morning with a sense of fatigue, as great as when he retired the night before.

Of all the chambers which are occupied by those who possess the most means, and those who most cultivate refinement of taste and manners, the chambers of *hotels* may be regarded as the worst, from their small size, their great number in proportion to the space, and the total absence of ventilation in them.

Now, this retention and concentration of the gaseous emanations of the lungs, the skin, etc., are, in general, as easily avoided as they are certainly injurious. There is scarcely a room in an ordinary dwelling whose atmosphere can not be, more or less, changed ; while there are many which may be readily ventilated, with little or no cost, and an opportunity given for an escape of the foul air of the room, sufficiently rapid to insure a complete avoidance of all danger of re-inhaling it.

Who that has passed a night on one of those floating
palaces, which have contributed, almost as much as the
natural scenery, to give a character to the Hudson river,
—and been obliged to occupy a berth or a settee in the
cabin below deck—has not most earnestly, in the morning, wished that the owners would adopt some method
of exhausting the foul air? Those who have never
been in that situation, can not realise the sickening sense
of oppression experienced in the morning, on awaken-
ing to the reality of having breathed the same air for
six or eight hours, with three hundred to four hundred
others, without any renewal whatever.

And yet the intelligent, sensitive, and delicate public,
which will not knowingly drink from the same glass as
another, nor permit a particle of dust to remain upon
its clothing any longer than it can possibly be brushed
off, will continue to crowd those sub-aqueous cellars,
sleep in those narrow boxes in treble tiers—(if sleep
the feverish, restless, semi-obliviousness can be called)—
will inhale, a score or more times, the air reeking from
the mouths of hundreds of others, and submit to the
disgusting and dangerous infliction without a murmur or
remonstrance; and this, too, when the engine which pro-
pels them along, affords the most powerful and cheapest
means known for complete ventilation. As an instance
of the utter indifference of the owners of these craft to
the genuine comfort of the passenger, it is related, that
the builders of the engine of the "Oregon," of New
York, when putting in the machinery, suggested that a
ventilating apparatus might easily be appended, so as to
keep all the apartments of the boat supplied with pure
air; but the wealthy proprietor contemptuously refused
the notion.

Such is the case, also, almost without exception, with
rail-cars and omnibuses,—into the latter of which, we

often see twelve, and occasionally fifteen or eighteen people crowded, with the windows and doors closed as tightly as possible. Now, an ordinary-sized omnibus can not contain more than two hundred and fifty cubic feet of air when empty; but when crowded with passengers, the actual amount of air must be reduced to at least one half, sometimes to one quarter, thus leaving only from three to ten cubic feet for the supply of each one. It is not possible to make more than one or two respirations, under these circumstances, without inhaling a portion of the breath of one's fellow-passengers, — the small crevices of the vehicle being utterly inadequate to a sufficient change of air. Nearly all this disgusting evil might be obviated by ventilating arrangements

6

CHAPTER VII.

Rationale of " Taking Cold," on emerging from a Crowded Room into the
Open Air.—Oxygen the Vital Element, and Carbonic Acid the fatal Element of Air.—Amount of Air required by each Person.—Different Estimates.—House of Commons.—Case of a Schoolhouse supposed.—Amount
of Solid Carbon thrown off from the Body.—Peculiar demand of the
Brain for Pure Air—especially in the Hours of Study.—Evil Effects of
School Atmosphere.—Illustration.

THE necessity of an abundant supply of oxygen, for
the maintenance of a vigorous condition of health, and
a *reactive energy* of the system, has been asserted in the
foregoing pages.   This, one of the cardinal points of the
philosophy of atmospheric influence, if clearly understood, will enable the reader to comprehend the reasoning by which it will now be attempted to be shown, why
it is, that, on emerging into the open air, after a continuance of a few hours in a crowded room, whether a lecture-room, church, ball-room, or school-room, there is
always so great a danger—to use the common phrase—
of "taking cold," in other words, of exciting an inflammation of some organ or tissue of the body.

This occurrence, so justly dreaded, yet so very common, is attributed, generally, to the *elevated temperature*
of the room, by which an excited action of the skin, and
a copious perspiration, are induced, the sudden suppres-
sion of which, and the consequent determination of the
blood from the surface of the body to the central organs,
throwing upon the latter a greater burden than they can
bear, excites in them an inflammation, whence other
diseases, more or less serious and severe, often result.

This is, indeed, as far as it goes, the explanation of the mode in which the effect is produced; but the reason why this effect should be produced, — why the mere assembling of people together, should be followed by such terrible results as we are often compelled to witness — why there should lurk in the path of duty, or instruction, no less than of pleasure, so venomous a poison, as we too often find developing itself in the human system, — the reason for all this lies deeper than the skin, and these effects are not to be accounted for by a change of temperature merely.

If the proposition is admitted, that the absorption of oxygen into, and the removal of carbon from, the system, are necessary to its energy and healthfulness, the converse proposition, that a deficient supply of oxygen, and the retention and accumulation of carbon will be productive of a depressed energy and tone, must also be admitted. The presence of carbonic acid in undue quantity, in the respired air, it has also been demonstrated, operates directly to impair the energy of the vital functions; even, when very abundant, to the total extinction of life. There is, moreover, in a crowded room, a diminished quantity of air, in consequence of the high temperature causing rarefaction, and the great amount of solid substances, which exclude an equal amount of air; — each piece of furniture and each individual, displacing of course, a bulk of the fluid equal to itself.

The combustion necessary for warming and lighting, also, is an additional source of abstraction of the vital properties of the atmosphere.

From these various causes, we find, in the area occupied by the company, in the first place a diminished amount of air, and, secondly, a rapid deterioration of it.

The two important conditions of the air, viz., the decrease of oxygen and the generation of carbonic acid, rapidly result, tending to produce the effects upon the system already adverted to, viz., an accumulation of carbon, and the inhalation of a poisonous gas.

Now the reverse of these circumstances is essential to the maintenance of a vigorous reactive energy, without which it is impossible for the system to sustain itself healthfully under the depressing influences to which it is continually subjected,—but with which, the variations of temperature, moisture, and the like, are calculated to act, within certain limits, rather as healthful stimuli to the different functions.

In a highly-heated and crowded room, therefore, the system is not only deprived, in a great degree, of the means necessary for its invigoration, but it is also subjected to circumstances which directly depress its vital powers, and render it unable to meet the attack of the cold air which it encounters on leaving the house. Both the nervous and circulatory functions of the skin are in an excited and active condition,—a double duty devolving upon this organ, to compensate for the deficient exercise of the functions of the lungs. Thus circumstanced, the sudden contraction of the cutaneous vessels by the cold air, drives an unusual amount of blood to the central organs, overwhelming them with its influx. In a healthy, vigorous condition, under ordinary circumstances, the internal organs, instead of being overcome by the sudden irruption, and succumbing under the shock, will be stimulated by it to a healthy reaction, and the whole system feel a genial and invigorating glow.

The system is, under the hypothesis, depressed by a want of its natural stimulus, oxygen; its reactive energy is greatly diminished, and it is unprepared to meet the emergency.

But with a full supply of oxygen, and a sufficiently rapid removal of the carbon, the condition of the various organs would be such as to enable them not only to meet the attack, but to be benefited by it.

Sudden changes of temperature, merely, in a healthy condition of body, do not necessarily cause disease, under common circumstances. It is said of the Russians, that a favorite exercise is to emerge from a hot bath and plunge in the snow; and with us, ablutions of cold water, by plunging or the shower-bath, in our hottest weather, are exceedingly grateful and invigorating. These vicissitudes are not more sudden, nor greater, than in the case under discussion; but there is a wide difference in the circumstances under which they are made.

Accumulations of carbonic acid, and other noxious gases, in crowded and heated apartments, are not unavoidable; and therefore, the depressing and unhealthful influences so commonly attendant upon the "assembling of ourselves together," are by no means inexorable. But well-devised systems of *Ventilation*, by discharging the room of its air, and supplying it with an equal amount from without, with a rapidity proportioned to the necessity of the case, will obviate the dangers otherwise imminent. Nothing else is needed to preserve the healthful tone of the system, than to remove the offending substances, and supply it duly with its proper aliment and stimulant.

With a sufficient means of maintaining its purity, the atmosphere of a crowded room would be innocuous,— both body and mind more vigorous and elastic,— and a most potent cause of disease and death happily obviated.

As oxygen is the vital element of air, so carbonic acid may be designated its fatal element—at least, when it exists in too large a proportion;* and though oxygen

---

*A certain proportion of carbonic acid is thought, by some, to be a necessary ingredient in the atmosphere; but when it exceeds one half per cent., all are agreed that its presence is injurious.

is indispensable to the maintenance of life, its activity in that capacity is far from being so great as that of carbonic acid in destroying vitality.

Dr. D. B. Reid has shown, by experiment, that it is not so much the deficiency of oxygen, as the presence of carbonic acid, in the air inspired, which impedes the aeration of the blood; and he has shown that an animal may be kept alive in a limited quantity of air, until nearly all its oxygen is exhausted, if an effectual provision be made for drawing off the carbonic acid as fast as it is generated.

The amount of air required by a human being, varies according to circumstances; the mature and robust requiring more than the weak, infant, or aged—the male more than the female. Also, under all circumstances, more is used during the day than at night—in health than in sickness—in a high temperature than a low—during muscular exercise than at rest—after a meal than when hungry—when the attention of the person experimented upon is drawn to the function of respiration, than when he is unconscious of its performance. These modifying circumstances, lately discovered by Prout, Edwards, and others, were, altogether or in part, overlooked by Black, Priestley, Lavoisier, Davy, and the earlier experimentalists, on this important point; and hence the discrepancy in their calculations, and the difficulty of coming to correct results at the present day. The point of greatest practical utility is not, however, disputed: when air contains above one half per cent. of carbonic acid, it may not be immediately, or rather palpably, injurious to the organism, but it is eventually so; while, on the other hand, if it contains above seven or eight per cent., it will prove suddenly fatal. According to some, three or four feet of pure air per minute is sufficient for a proper aeration of the blood. Others, though they admit that this quantity might possibly be endured for a considerable time, without any well-defined deterioration of constitution, contend that this circumstance is no proof of its sufficiency, and advise at least *ten cubic feet per minute for each individual.* It was observed in the British House of Commons, that any less than ten feet was soon noticeable on the health of the members; and they even expressed feelings of discomfort, in a high temperature, with any less than forty or fifty. According to the most reliable experiments and calculations, it is found that ten cubic feet is a fair standard to test the sufficiency of an atmosphere inhaled; as no smaller quantity is capable of removing all doubts as to the latent and eventual evils of a deficiency.

Let us suppose the case of a school-room, containing 10,000 cubic feet $(50 \times 20 \times 10)$ of perfectly pure air (if such there be), with two hundred pupils. To each of them will be allowed ten cubic feet of air per minute. To avoid every chance of exaggeration, and to adapt the calculation to age and size, no deduction will be made for the pupils themselves, or for their seats, desks, furniture, books, &c., all of which substances do displace an equal bulk of air, and by so much reduce the quantity actually in the room.

According to these premises, there would be fifty feet for each pupil; and supposing that there existed no communication with the external air (which would generally be the case if the doors and windows were closely shut), the air of the room would be rendered unfit for respiration by the carbonic acid alone, without including the other exhalations, *in just five minutes.* Or in other words, the pupils would, at the end of five minutes, begin to inhale, again and again, the excrementitious matter from their own and one another's bodies. Again, suppose, with Liebig, that ten ounces of solid carbon would be excreted from each of their bodies in twenty-four hours, — at the end of one hour, eighty-four ounces, or seven pounds troy, of this poison, would be held in solution in the air of the room, and be constantly going the round of the circulation, sowing the seeds of death. These seven pounds of carbon would, in an hour, form one hundred and seventy-six cubic feet of carbonic acid, which implies the removal of one hundred and eighty feet of oxygen.   And as the oxygen originally amounted to (as 80 : 20 :: 10,000 : 2500) twenty-five hundred cubic feet, this gas would (supposing the circumstances favorable for its combination with carbon) be entirely exhausted in fourteen or fifteen hours.   But as the accumulation of carbon in the atmosphere of the room, impedes the excretion of more from the beginning, and as this substance is as fatal to life when retained as when inhaled, many of the pupils would not be living, a long time before the entire removal of the oxygen.

It may be objected that cases such as the above seldom occur.—Admitted; but this depends upon the fact, that there are generally broken panes,* keyholes, or crevices of some kind, through which there is an ingress for the fresh, and an exit for the impure, air; and it is true, that when there is a certain amount of ventilation, there is a limit to the concentration of carbonic acid.   This circumstance, however, instead of divesting impure air of its terrors, in reality enhances them, as the inmates are thus lulled into a false security, whose deceptiveness is only discovered, if it ever is, when the seeds of disease which have been thus sown, germinate and ripen into fatal maturity.

There are certain physiological truths which have a most important connexion with the subject of ventilation,

---

* How many lives have broken panes been the means of saving, as well as destroying!

when considered in relation to the functions of the Brain.

The first of these truths is, that the brain, though its weight is only *one fortieth* of that of the whole body, yet it is estimated to receive *one fifth* of all the blood which flows from the heart. In proportion to its bulk, its arteries are more numerous, and larger, than any other.

The reason for this most extraordinary distinction, is found in the peculiar character of its duties. It is the immediate seat of the mind; it never sleeps; as the organ of thought, it is ever at work: while the organs of digestion, of motion, and others, are in repose, and obtaining a renewal of strength, it is in action, superintending, as it were, the performance of all the others, and has no rest.

The next fact to be noticed in this connexion is, that it is especially in the *hours of study*, when the brain works hardest, it requires the blood with which it is furnished to be decarbonized to the utmost degree. It was the opinion of the celebrated physiologist Boerhaave, that the blood sent to the brain is more aerated than any other, an opinion probably formed from the fact that it is sent to it sooner and more directly, after passing through the lungs.

In addition to these physiological truths, we have, in proof of the greater necessity of supplying the brain with pure blood, the pathological fact of the greater and more immediate liability of this organ to disease, by the inhalation of impure air. Its effects are *first* seen upon the mental and other faculties directly dependent on this organ, and then through it upon other functions. Sudden and fatal results are well known to ensue from the respiration of carbonic acid gas in a more concentrated form, but serious pathological effects are scarcely less certain, though they may be less immediate, when this noxious gas is breathed in the more diluted form, in which it is found in long-used and pent-up apartments.

Among the effects produced by remaining in an impure atmosphere, there is an almost immediate one to which the attention of teachers, and all concerned in the care of schools, should be constantly drawn; it is, that condition of listlessness, languor, and irritability, so often observed in both pupils and teachers. Irritability of the nervous system, as well as dullness of the intellect, is unquestionably the direct result of a want of pure air. The vital energies of the pupil are more or less prostrated by it— he becomes restless and indisposed to attend to his books and rules—his mind wanders from his studies—and he unavoidably seeks relief for the natural appetite for air, in disorderly actions which call for reprimand from his teacher, who, from the same cause, is perhaps in the same irritable and unhealthy condition of mind and body, which must also find a vent some how and upon some thing. Thus irritability grows to irritation, until it becomes a question of serious import, how far, as a corrective, or, rather, preventive, of this evil, pure air would serve in substitution for the ferule, and whether the natural stimulation of oxygen would not be more easy of application and more sure of effect, than the artificial sedative of the strap.

It has fallen to the lot of the writer to see many instances of the injurious influence of the foul air of school-rooms, both private and public, on the health of pupils, even to fatal terminations. He has seen children grow pale and thin, and gradually droop and sicken, without any cause visible to the parents, who, in their grief, have attributed all to the dispensation of an inscrutable Providence, without a thought of the true source of the calamity, until it has been (alas, too late!) pointed out to them. It were easy to cite, from actual experi-

ence, cases of sickness and death of pupils, the com-
mencements of which were undoubtedly laid in the places
which, of all others, should be least obnoxious to the
charge; the most unhappy feature of which is, that the
teachers themselves are, in too many instances, ignorant
of the true merits of pure air, and unwilling to admit
the humiliating fact, so easily demonstrated, that the
atmosphere of their school-rooms is offensive and dangerous.

The following, however, quoted from an official docu-
ment,* will suffice to exhibit the subject in its true
light :—

" Before dismissing this subject, I will refer to a
school which I visited during the winter of 1841–'2, in
which the magnitude of the evil under consideration was
clearly developed. Five of the citizens of the district
attended me in my visit to the school. We arrived at
the schoolhouse about the middle of the afternoon. It
was a close, new house, eighteen by twenty-four feet on
the ground. There were present forty-three scholars,
the teacher, five patrons, and myself, making fifty in all.
Immediately after entering the schoolhouse, one of the
trustees remarked to me, ' I believe our schoolhouse is
too tight to be healthy.' I made no reply, but secretly
resolved, that I would sacrifice my comfort for the remainder of the afternoon, and hazard my health, and my
life, even, to test the accuracy of the opinion I had entertained on this important subject. I marked the unea-
siness and dullness of all present, and especially of the
patrons, who had been accustomed to breathe a purer
atmosphere. School continued an hour and a half, at
the close of which I was invited to make some remarks.
I arose to do so, but was unable to proceed, till I opened

* Annual Report of Ira Mayhew, Superintendent of Public Instruction
of the State of Michigan, for the year 1847.

the outer door, and snuffed a few times, the purer air
without. When I had partially recovered my wonted
vigor, I observed, with delight, the renovating influence
of the current of air that entered the door, mingling
with and gradually displacing the fluid poison that filled
the room, and was about to do the work of death. It
seemed as though I were standing at the mouth of a
huge sepulchre, in which the dead were being restored
to life. After a short pause, I proceeded with a few remarks, chiefly, however, on the subject of respiration
and ventilation. The trustees, who had just tested their
accuracy and bearing upon their comfort and health,
resolved immediately to provide for ventilation according to the suggestions about to be given. When I next
heard from the neighborhood, their arrangements were
effected. Before leaving the house on that occasion, I
was informed an evening meeting had been attended
there the preceding week, which they were obliged to
dismiss before the ordinary exercises were concluded,
because, as they said, " We all got sick, and the candles
went almost out." Little did they realize, probably, that
the light of life became just as nearly extinct as did the
candles. Had they remained there a little longer, both
would have gone out together, and there would have
been reacted the memorable tragedy of the *black hole* in
Calcutta, into which were thrust a garrison of one hundred and forty-six persons, one hundred and twenty-three
of whom perished miserably in a few hours, being suffocated by the confined air."

CHAPTER VIII.

EFFECTS OF VITIATED AIR UPON THE HUMAN SYSTEM.

Impure Air one of the Scourges of Mankind.—No Age or Sex Exempt.—
Pestilential Winds.—Maladies from preventible Causes.—Carbonic
Oxide Gas.—Carburetted Hydrogen.—Two Species of Aerial Poison.—
Gaseous Compounds of Sulphur and Ammonia.—Causes of Fever.—
Opinion of F. Southwood Smith, M. D. ; of Dr. Arnott ; of Dr. Emerson.
—Effects of Indoor Labor on the Health—Examples.—Epidemic stop-
ped by Ventilation.—" Black Hole of Calcutta "—Further Illustrations
from E. Chadwick.—Dr. Rush, and the Yellow Fever in Philadelphia.
—Prudence of the Chinese —Cleanliness contributive to Health.—Ro-
man Enterprise.—Cloacæ.—Sanatory Movements in Turkey and Egypt.
—Unfavorable Circumstances attending Ships, greatly Remediable.—Il-
lustrative Anecdote.—Awful Catastrophe.—Child-Bed Fever.—Exam-
ination of Dr. Rigby.—Influence of Foul Air in Producing and of Pure
Air in Preventing it.—Peculiar Odor of Bedrooms.—Other Contagious
Viri communicated through the Atmosphere ; as of Small Pox, Measles,
Scarlet Fever, &c.—Secondary Influence of Miasmata on the Consti-
tution.—Further Observations of Dr. T. S. Smith.—Diseases of the
Digestive Organs.—Particular Influence of Bad Air on Mothers and
Children.—Its Influence not confined to the Physical Functions ; but ex-
tends to the Mental Faculties.—Examples.

In the foregoing pages, an attempt has been made to
explain the composition of atmospheric air, in its pure
and vitiated states ;—the machinery which is employed by
Nature, when unimpeded in her operations, to vivify, by
means of oxygen, the circulating fluid ;—and the uniformly injurious consequences, resulting to organic life, from

7

respiring impure or contaminated air. It has also been demonstrated, in a general manner, that, while the air, in its purity, contains, within itself, the elements of life, and health, and corporeal, and mental energy: it is in its vitiated state, pregnant with the hidden causes of physical, moral, and social degeneracy and decay. It now remains to detail, more minutely, the effects of the inhalation of air, mixed with chemical or mechanical impurities, on the human constitution, as exhibited in the consequent diseased conditions of both body and mind. Volumes might be profitably filled with this important subject, as impure air is the direct cause of very many, and an aggravation of *all* the diseases incident to the human frame; but it would be incompatible with the limits assigned to the present work, to aim at a full investigation of all the evils, referrible to partial or complete derangements of the function of respiration.

Impure air is, indeed, one of the scourges of mankind. No age or sex is exempted from its influences, but especially are they obnoxious to its evils who have adopted, or complied with, the modern ideas of civilization, and refinement—and this prime and ever-operating cause of disease, depopulation, and premature mortality has existed in its various modifications, and produced its deleterious effects, in a greater or less degree at all times, and in all countries and climates.

Some of the vitiated conditions of the atmosphere depend, it must be acknowledged, on causes, over which mankind have, as yet, no control: such as the *simoom, sirocco, harmattan,* and other poisonous and pestilential winds of eastern countries; as also the conditions which produce plagues, and many contagious, endemic and epidemic diseases, which up to the present time, have baffled human investigation; but it may be fully shown, as a fact (at which influential and scientific men may well blush), *that at least one half of the maladies daily hurrying their victims to untimely graves, arise from easily understood and preventible causes.*

No doubt great uncertainties have prevailed, and still prevail, respecting the origin of diseases from certain gases, vapors, and mechanical impurities, floating through the air; but speculation will be avoided as much as possible and well-ascertained facts, and the opinions of eminent men founded on facts, only, will be depended on in the following pages.

It has already been explained that carbonic acid gas, when inspired, is a fertile source of disease, and even death. Other compounds of carbon are often present in the atmosphere, and are equally deleterious, and morbific, though generally slower in their operation. One or two instances will suffice;—Sir Humphry Davy took three inspirations of carbonic oxide,* mixed with about one fourth of common air; the effect was a temporary loss of sensation, which was succeeded by giddiness, sickness, acute pains in different parts of the body, and extreme debility; some days elapsed before he completely recovered.—Mr. Witter of Dublin fell down, apoplectic, while breathing this gas, but was restored by the inhalation of oxygen (Phil. Mag., vol. 43). In chambers, especially those that are ill-ventilated, where anthracite coal is burning, it is often present in considerable quantities, and may be seen burning in a dark blue flame on the surface of the fire. It is, though combustible, a non-supporter of combustion or of life, hence it is impossible to light a paper on the top of an anthracite fire.

Carburetted hydrogen gas, a compound of carbon and hydrogen, containing no oxygen, is also highly fatal to

* A combination of oxygen and carbon, containing one proportion less of oxygen, than carbonic acid gas.

animal life.   It is the "*choke-damp*" or "*fire-damp*" that
has poisoned so many miners: and may possibly be generated in damp cellars, and underground basements
(from which the fresh air has been excluded) to such an
extent as gradually to impair the constitution of those
subjected to it.   It also constitutes an effluvium from the
mud of stagnant pools, open sewers, and ditches, "and to
procure it," says Dr. Ure, " we have only to fill a wide-
mouthed vial with water, and inverting it in the ditch,
stir the bottom with a stick.   Gas rises into the goblet."
But of all morbific agents in the production of disease,
perhaps the compounds of sulphur are most to be dreaded, because they are least easily to be guarded against.
When coal containing sulphur (and it is rarely found
without it), is burned, it not only forms with oxygen,
carbonic acid, but also by the sulphur combining with
the oxygen of the air—*sulphurous acid*, which, if not very
largely diluted by fresh air, will be immediately followed
by irritation of the air passages, inflammation of the
lungs, and even, if inhaled in considerable quantity,
spasmodic contractions of the windpipe, and occasionally
suffocation.

*Writers on pestilence note two distinct species of virus,
applied to the body through the medium of the air*, viz.:
1st, that arising from the putrefaction, or decomposition
of dead animal or vegetable matter: as the exhalations
of marshes, sewers, graveyards, bogs, uncultivated or
undrained places, the accumulation of filth in cities,
houses, &c.; 2d, effluvia generated by the decomposition
of the natural exhalations, and excretions of the human
body, accumulated, and confined in ill-ventilated habitations.—The first has been called *marsh miasm*, and is
supposed on good grounds to give rise to yellow, remittent,
bilious, and intermittent fevers, dysentery, and perhaps
also cholera.—The second species, sometimes termed the

typhoid miasm, usually gives origin to common typhus, and low nervous fevers. A variety of opinion exists as to the nature of these miasms. Some affirm that the disorders caused by the first-named variety are not in any degree " dependent on the predominance of nitrogen, of carburetted hydrogen, of ammonia, of nitrous oxide, &c., in the air," while many others, e. g. Hooper (*Med. Dicty.*, article *Contagion*), after admitting that the "chemical nature of all these poisonous effluvia is little understood," goes on to state that " they *undoubtedly* consist of *hydrogen* united with sulphur, phosporus, carbon, and nitrogen, in unknown proportions and unknown states of combination." Later observations would tend to confirm the last opinion. Liebig has succeeded in detecting ammonia in the atmosphere, and by a series of carefully-conducted experiments, Dr. Gardner of Hampden Sydney college, has well nigh established the identity of *malaria* with sulphuretted hydrogen. These opinions are held by the best authorities that could be cited, and on the whole it would appear that *sulphuret of ammonia* is the morbific agent exciting typhus fever, *sulphuretted hydrogen* being the pestilential virus producing yellow-fever, and the bilious remittents, and agues of tropical climates. It is quite probable however, that both miasms when acting at the same time, produce a disease of a new type. Prof. Smith, of New York, says, " Let us suppose the circumstances in which typhus originates to occur in summer, such as the crowding of individuals into small apartments badly ventilated, and rendered offensive by personal and domestic filth; these causes would obviously produce typhus in its ordinary form. But suppose there exist at the same time those exhalations which occasion plague and yellow-fever or remittent and intermittent fevers; under such circumstances we would not expect to see any one of those diseases fully and distinctly formed, but a

7*

disease of a new and modified character. It is therefore beyond probability, that a few deleterious gases are quite sufficient to produce an infinite variety of pestilential and contagious maladies."

It is easy to account for the prevalence of these diseases, in the middle and torrid regions of the earth, where there is a superabundant quantity of dead animal and vegetable matter, and where heat and moisture, the two necessary agents for its decomposition, are always present to a greater or less extent. Dr. Carmichael Smith discovered that the vapors of nitrous acid neutralize and render harmless the typhus miasm, which he ascertained to be sulphuret of ammonia, and on the utility of this discovery being duly tested and confirmed, a sum of £5000 was voted to him, by the British parliament, as a national donation.*

A few quotations will be made to show the opinions of men who have given their attention to this important subject, and who are well qualified to estimate the influence of atmospheric impurities and want of ventilation in the production of febrile and other malarious diseases. " I conceive the immediate and direct cause of fever to be, a poison generated by the decomposition of animal and vegetable matters. It is only by a good and general sewerage, that the animal and vegetable refuse which there must always be where there are human beings, and the quantity of which must of course be great, in pro-

---

* This method is still used, with the best results, in disinfecting ships, jails. hospitals, &c., and clothes that may have been imbued with the poison The gas is readily obtained by pouring oil of vitriol, or sulphuric acid, on an equal weight of powdered nitre. in a cup, placed on a heated iron plate, stove, &c. It is to be cautiously stirred, and the first fumes carefully avoided. Chlorine has also been efficaciously used as a disinfecting agent. It is also easily obtained—chloride of lime is to be put into a shallow vessel, and made into a paste with water, and spread thinly over the bottom of the vessel. Sulphuric acid, diluted with water, is then poured over it, and chlorine gas in large quantities is rapidly evolved.

portion to the number of persons that are congregated together, and therefore must always be largest in the largest towns and in the most densely-populated parts of those towns, can be removed before putrefaction takes place, and consequently the poison of fever is matured and diffused. Hence the rapid and complete removal of this refuse matter, which it is the object of sewerage to effect, is the primary and fundamental means of preventing the production of fever; without this all other precautions must be in vain; and next in importance to this is ventilation; both because currents of air are to the poisonous gases when generated, what the sewers are to the solid matters from which the gases are produced— that is, the great means of carrying them off; and because the free admixture of pure air with poisonous gases, by diluting them, renders them innoxious."—*T. Southwood Smith, M. D.*

" Our inquiries give us the conviction that the immediate and chief cause of many of the diseases which impair the bodily and mental health of the people, and bring a considerable portion prematurely to the grave, is the poison of *atmospheric impurity*, arising from the accumulation in and around their dwellings, of the decomposing remnants of the substances used for food, and in their arts, and of the impurities given out from their own bodies."—" If you allow the sources of aerial impurity to exist in or around dwellings, you are poisoning the people; and while many may die at early ages of fevers and other acute diseases, the remainder will have their health impaired and their lives shortened. An unhealthy race will have arisen in consequence of the great defect. . . . They may tell their medical man, when he makes any representation to them on the subject (ventilation) that ' ventilation is a hobby of his and that hitherto people have got on very well without attending to it.' If they hear of such occurrences as that in the first American war, of two thousand British seamen dying in one fleet from fever and want of ventilation, it is not their case, and they can not understand it."—*Dr. Arnott, to the " Commissioners for inquiring into the state of large towns and populous districts in England."*

Notwithstanding the great numbers of those who die annually of cholera, we feel ourselves warranted in asserting that deaths from this disease are rare in houses with large and well-aired apartments.

" It is common to attribute the greater mortality known to take place under ordinary circumstances in large towns, among the poorer classes, chiefly to meager or unwholesome food, and immoderate indulgence in strong liquors. But in this country, where for a part of the year we are subjected to a degree of heat little, if at all, below that of the tropics, the influence of both these causes in the production of disease is, in our opinion, insignificant, when compared to that of breathing air that has been previously respired, and which moreover is commonly charged with animal and vegetable effluvia. That the same diet and habits of life in the country, or small towns, would not be attended with a degree of sickness and mortality corresponding to that found in the crowded portions of large towns, is, we think, beyond a doubt." —*Dr. Governeur Emerson, on the Medical Statistics of Philadelphia.*

Dr. Emerson's opinion is confirmed in other quarters. The following corroborations are taken from Dr. Arnott:

" In Spitalfields, London, a severe epidemic broke out in a time of comparatively full employment. Subsequently the employment diminished, so that not more than one half the handloom weavers [who make up almost all the population] were at work. The medical officer of the district found that immediately after the diminution of employment there was a decrease of fever patients from eight hundred to two hundred and fifty. He states that ' The greatest number of fever cases we have is of persons who fall ill during the time they are in employment. I think they are more attacked when in work, when the windows are closed, and there is no ventilation; — when they are out of work they are more out of doors, looking after work — more in the open air; and that very exercise may be the means of keeping them in health.' . . . In May, 1832, there was an almost entire cessation of work at Paisley [a manufacturing town in Scotland] so extensive, that extraordinary means were taken, by general subscriptions, and with the aid of the government, to relieve the distress. At that precise time, the medical men having the charge of the fever hospital were surprised by an extraordinary diminution in the number of cases of fever. There were during that month just one eighth less than the average during five preceding years. But the demand for goods and labor subsequently returned, so that the whole population was again employed, and warehouses were cleared of goods that had not been empty for ten years before. In this restored state of the labor-market, a new epidemic broke out."

Many instances are on record where the progress of an epidemic has been suddenly stopped by ventilation. " When I visited Glasgow," says Dr. Arnott, " with Mr. Chadwick, there was described to us one vast lodging house, in connexion with a manufactory there, in which formerly fever constantly prevailed, but where, by making an opening from the top of each room through a channel of communication to an air-pump, common to all the channels, the disease had disappeared altogether. The supply of pure air obtained by that mode of ventilation, was sufficient to dilute the cause of the disease, so that it became powerless."

In the famous "black hole" of Calcutta, one hundred and forty-six Englishmen were shut up at night by order of Surajah Dowlah, only twenty-three of whom were found alive in the morning. In this case, as they had not more than four or five thousand cubic feet of air, and as, for healthful purposes, there are required at least three hundred cubic feet for each man, many of them must have been almost immediately poisoned by the large volume of carbonic acid gas emitted from their lungs. This volume of course diminished as they died, the oxygen decreased less rapidly, and thus a remnant was left. But these also must have received a highly concentrated dose of the ammoniacal effluvia arising from the putrifying exhalations of their bodies. Accordingly, they are said *" to have been attacked with a fever analogous to typhus."*

Besides the above facts, thousands of instances could be adduced to show that when the alleged causes of fever, viz., deficient ventilation and impure air, were removed, fever disappeared also. Mr. Chadwick, in his report on the sanatory condition of the laboring classes in Great Britain, says " there was in Glasgow," previously to his visit to that city, "attached to one of the factories, an assemblage of dwellings for the work people, called from its mode of construction, and the crowd collected in it, *' the barracks.'* This building contained five hundred persons ; every room contained one family. The consequences of this crowding of the apartments, which were badly ventilated, and the filth, were, that fever was scarcely ever absent from the building. There were sometimes as many as seven cases in one day, and in the last two months of 1831 there were fifty-seven cases in the building. All attempts to induce the inmates to ventilate their rooms were ineffectual, and the proprietors of the work, on the recommendation of Mr. Fleming, a surgeon of the district, fixed a simple tin tube, of two inches diameter, the extremity of which was inserted into the chimney of the factory furnace. By the perpetual draught thus produced upon the atmosphere of each room, the inmates were *compelled*, whether they would or no, to breathe pure air. The effect was, that during the ensuing eight years fever was scarcely known in the place. The cost of remedies previously applied in the public hospitals, to the fever cases continually produced, as described in ' the barracks,' was stated by Dr. Cowan to have afforded a striking contrast to the cost of the means of prevention." Before the days of Howard (deservedly called "the good") jail fever existed almost constantly, in all the jails of Europe. At present, at least one fourth of them are somewhat better ventilated, and it is notorious that there is not one fourth the amount of fever now in those institutions, that formerly existed. It would seem from the statement of Dr. Rush, that yellow fever in Philadelphia has yielded to the progress of sanatory reform. "And Philadelphia must admit," says Doctor Rush, " the unwelcome truth, sooner or later, that the yellow fever is engendered in her own bowels; or she must renounce her character for knowledge and policy, and perhaps with it, her existence, as a commercial city." However, the cleanliness and ventilation of Philadelphia (though like those wholesome measures in all large towns, still defective) present a strong contrast, with her sanatory condition at the time when Dr. Rush made his observation; and it is to be presumed that her " knowledge and " policy" have fortunately averted the calamities referred to, by adopting the measure the " Sydenham of America" has suggested.

It might be supposed at first thought, that China and

Japan would be frequently ravaged with fever, the inhabitants being so much crowded, and the cities so populous. But such is not the case, and the Chinese are proverbially exempt from fever. Such is the value laid on manure, and the animal and vegetable filth of towns, that these substances are promptly carried away, and applied to their proper uses, before their precious gases escape ; and thus those pestilential effluvia, which in other countries destroy life, are here turned into the means of supporting it. But, in this country, with its boasted civilization, so much indifference prevails on this point, that we may often see a farmer, who stands high in the scale of intelligence, mortified at the parching influence of a hot season on his crops, but without ever bestowing a sigh on the bright gold, which under the form of ammonia, is constantly making its escape from the farmsteading, and perchance, communicating disease and death to his family or his cattle.

Mankind appear to have soon discovered that cleanliness contributed to their health, and plague and pestilence seem to have been considerably under the control of their sanatory measures ; otherwise cleanliness would not have constituted a part of their religion. It is almost unnecessary to refer to the scrupulous regard to cleanliness, inculcated in the laws of Moses. Similar laws prevailed in Egypt and Greece. *Cloacæ,* or sewers, on a magnificent scale, were commenced shortly after the foundation of the Roman city. Their object was "to remove all filth, and ordure, which in a great capital too often breed pestilence and diseases." A brief description from Lempriere (Classical Dictionary) will give some idea of the enterprise of the ancient Romans in this important branch of civilization. " The *cloacæ* were large receptacles, for the filth and dung of the whole city. They were begun by Tarquin, the fifth king of Rome, and finished by his grandson, Tarquin *the proud*, about six hundred years before the Christian era. They were built under the city, and the arches were so high that according to Procopius, a man on horseback might ride through them, even in the ordinary course of the channel, and a wain, loaded with hay, might pass, and vessels sail in them. There were in the streets, at proper distances, openings for the admission of dirty water, or any other filth, which persons were appointed always to remove, and also to keep the cloacæ clean. The principal sewer, now existing, with which the rest communicated, was called the *cloca maxima* (great sewer), and was principally the work of the younger Tarquin. The cloacæ were at first carried through the streets, but from the want of regularity in building the city, after it was burned by the Gauls, they, in many places, passed under private houses. The cleaning of the cloacæ was the more easily effected by means of the declivity of the ground, and the plenty of water with which the city was supplied. Under the republic, certain officers, called *censors*, and who had other duties to perform, had charge of them ; but under the emperors regular *curators* were appointed, and a tax was imposed, for keeping them in repair."

The Romans were also convinced, that the marshes, in the neighborhood of the city, were very unwholesome ; and they took incredible pains, to render their city and territory healthful, by draining off all stagnant waters. Accordingly, Livy informs us that Cethegus, one of the consuls about five hundred and seventy-two years after the founding of the city, drained the famous Pontine marshes, and converted them into cultivable land. The Appian way, another great work of the ancient Romans, ran through marshes south of the city, that can not now be even approached. But in modern Italy, the energy

8

of their ancestors has departed, and malaria has pro-
gressed with fatal malignancy.*

Ancient Egypt was alike the nursery of the plague,
and the fine arts. The people, however, learned by experience to mitigate its attacks, and plague was on the
decline until the subjugation of the country by the Turks,
whose habits of living are said to have revived it.—*Han-
cock on Pestilence*, p. 289. Lately, however, in Turkey,
the government is encouraging sanatory measures, and
even in Egypt, where stagnant water, holding animal
and vegetable impurities in solution, is the main dependence of the people, the necessity of drainage and sanatory
laws has not been overlooked ; and these measures are
evidently attended with success.

Ships have always been miserably circumstanced, for
want of proper ventilation ; their peculiar structure preventing, in some measure, the adoption of efficient means.
To economize space, it was formerly the custom of the
masters of ships, engaged in the slave-trade, to cram between decks, without regard to ventilation, as many of
their miserable captives as could sit or lie ; and from the
natural activity of their exhalent systems, and especially
the copious secretion of the skin, a miasm was soon
generated, and very frequently one half, and sometimes
almost all, their number, fell a prey to typhus. Self-
interest, in a short time, administered the remedy that
humanity had denied, and slave importers have very
shrewdly taken the lead in ship ventilation. Even brutes
(because they have owners) are often treated with more
humanity than human beings themselves. On this principle, emigrants are usually deprived of the benefits of
ventilation, and legal enactments have, in most instances,

---

* Rome, once the mistress and wonder of the world, seems destined to
destruction by malaria, which is making its annual encroachments on the
city. M'Culloch thus describes modern Italy : " A land whose fragrant
breezes are poison, and the dews of whose summer evenings are death."

failed to reach the evil.   The following will suffice as an exhibition of the disregard of many in authority, of the comfort and safety of emigrant passengers.

During the last summer (1848), fever broke out on board a British emigrant ship, bound to New York, and on the surgeon representing to the captain the necessity of making a small opening through the deck, to carry the vitiated air up behind the forecastle, and thus ventilate the part of the ship where all the patients lay, he very decidedly declined "*injuring the ship ;*" and when one of the patients died, did not betray any observable qualms of conscience.   But his canary-bird, whose cage hung in the cabin, enjoyed daily a current of fresh air, except in wet weather, when the cabin passengers all but monopolized the fresh air, and deprived poor Dickey of his share of the oxygen, which made him very stupid, and put a full stop to his melodies.   His master, however, soon discovered the true nature of his complaint, and suddenly seemed to understand and appreciate the principles of ventilation, which he forthwith reduced to practice, by breaking open the cabin window.

The following awful catastrophe is related by Trotter, in his "View of the Nervous Temperament," and serves to illustrate the combined effects of self-interest and ignorance in connexion with this subject: "In 1797–'8, a small passage vessel belonging to Southampton, had on board *seventy* men, women, and children, coming from Jersey, among whom were many soldiers and their families.   It began to blow fresh breezes, and for the safety of his sloop, the master laid the hatches over and covered them with a tarpaulin, which he battened down for better security.   When the vessel came within the isle of Wight, the hatches were opened, but dreadful to be told! *the whole of the passengers were found dead!!!* The master, who did all (?) this through ignorance of the effects of *foul air*, became mad, and died soon after."

Only another species of febrile complaint will at present be noticed, but it is one which is perhaps more under the control of ventilation; and more dependent on the impurity of the air, than any yet mentioned, and which has especial claims on the attention of the patrons of benevolent institutions, viz.: child-bed fever. This formidable complaint very seldom makes its appearance in well-ventilated apartments. The answers of Dr. Edward Rigby to the commissioners, before alluded to, will throw some light on the connexion between such diseases and atmospheric impurities. We shall make a few quotations:—

"E. RIGBY, M. D., EXAMINED.

"Are you senior physician to the general lying-in hospital, Lambeth [London]?"—"I am."

"How long have you been a medical officer to that institution?"—"Since 1832 [12 years]."

"It may be presumed, that a lying-in hospital, from the peculiar susceptibility of the patients, is a place in which the effects of atmospheric impurities or miasma, would be more strikingly manifested, than with any other class?" —"Yes—the circumstances being the same in both cases —their effects would be more immediately manifest on such patients than upon any other class. From the various circumstances connected with the puerperal state, few patients render the surrounding air impure from animal effluvia more rapidly, than lying-in women, fever cases, perhaps, excepted."

"In the management of the hospital, were any difficulties encountered, either from the locality of the building, defective state of the house-drains, or adjoining sewers, or from deficient internal ventilation?"—"The hospital was seldom free, for any length of time, from puerperal fever, occasionally producing frightful ravages, and requiring the building, every now and then, to be closed. After the greatest attention had been paid to cleanliness, in every respect, the wards left open night and day for weeks, fumigated, the walls lined and painted, the beds thoroughly cleaned, fumigated, repaired, and frequently renewed, and the most scrupulous attention paid to cleanliness, the fever reappeared on some occasions, *immediately* on the hospital being reopened. This circumstance made us look to external causes, when we ascertained that in the immediate vicinity of the hospital, there were upward of fifteen hundred feet of open ditches, receiving the drainage of the poor and dense population of the neighborhood, one of the ditches being not more than thirty feet from the walls of the building. It was black and stagnant, and in constant ebullition from the disengagement of gas. After great difficulty and trouble, the hospital having to bear a large proportion of the expense, the commissioners of sewers were induced, though with much reluctance, to have a portion of these ditches cleaned and properly arched over; an immense quantity of black pestilential mud was excavated, but instead of being removed, it was spread over the adjoining ground. At that time the hospital was free from disease, but two cases of puerperal fever occurred within twenty-four hours after this unjustifiable act."

"Had you still cases of fever?"—"Puerperal fever still continued to make its appearance, from time to time, and occasionally with great severity. As the physicians were dissatisfied with the existing means for ventilating the wards, to such an extent as could be done with safety to the patients, and as it was found that unless quickly changed, the air became speedily loaded with effluvia, it was deemed advisable, in April, 1842, to adopt Dr. Reid's plan of ventilation; and accordingly a large sum

8*

was expended in the necessary alterations. When this new plan came into operation, much opposition was experienced by the female attendants, and great difficulty in preventing them from closing the different valves for admitting fresh and emitting foul air. In November, 1842, during a moist and unusually warm state of the atmosphere, for that season of the year, I found on visiting the hospital, one evening, that the air of one ward which had its full number of patients, all of whom had been recently delivered, was exceedingly close and oppressive, and the thermometer at seventy-five degrees, and it was stated to have been even so high as seventy-eight degrees; the air had a decidedly sour smell, and was evidently loaded with effluvia. This improper state of things had been produced by closing the valves and cutting off the ventilations in defiance of my strict orders to the contrary. I strongly remonstrated, declaring that puerperal fever would appear within twenty-four hours. In eighteen hours' time, I was called to see a woman with symptoms of the disease in that ward; she died, and several other women in the same ward were also attacked, but if I recollect rightly, recovered. The hospital continued in an unhealthy state until the following spring, when on finding (Feb. 1843), that water rose at times in the bottom of the shaft, where the fire is placed for producing the current of air, Dr. Reid carefully analysed some of it, and declared his conviction that it must have proceeded from some obstructed drain in the neighborhood. The entire drainage of the building was thoroughly examined and it was then ascertained the main drain was entirely blocked up by two logs of wood. The whole basement was flooded with every description of decomposing impurities, and it was impossible to tell how long this state of matters had existed. The whole ground must have been saturated with impurities to an extreme extent. In July, two of my own pupils became house-surgeons to the establishment; gentlemen in whom I placed the fullest confidence and who carried out my orders respecting the ventilation of the wards, in spite of much opposition and personal annoyance. From that moment we have not had a case of puerperal fever; the patients have been admitted broken down by poverty and misery; severe and dangerous labors have occurred among them, and there has been every possible variety of weather, but up to the present time since July, there has not occurred the slightest trace of puerperal fever."

"What is the nature of puerperal fever?"—"It is of the same class of diseases as the plague, yellow-fever, and the putrid marsh intermittents of tropical climates, &c.; diseases which essentially depend on a vitiated state of the blood, arising from the introduction of some (usually animal) poison into the circulating current."

"Is it communicable in the same way as the diseases to which you have alluded?"—"It is;—it may, in the first instance, be generated, under the ordinary circumstances which are known to favor the production of typhoid fevers; it may be propagated by contact; and it may become infectious, from the air being charged with effluvia, emanating from the patient, or her discharges. On this latter point I would, with permission, quote a passage from a work of my own, on these subjects: 'The lungs afford a ready and ample means by which effluvia may be conveyed into the circulating current, and enables us to account for the fact adduced by Dr. Stevens, that in situations favorable to the production of fevers, the blood is frequently found in a very unhealthy state, even before the outbreak of the disease itself."

Dr. Rigby goes on to say: "I have every reason to believe, that in a large majority of cases, the ventilation of private houses is very inferior to that of our large hospitals, more particularly as regards the effluvia from drains, &c. The arrangements also for ventilating the sleeping rooms, especially the servant's bedrooms, are very defective; the peculiar close disagreeable smell of the latter chambers, must be familiar to all."

We may here add that this peculiar *bedroomy* odor is not, as Dr. Rigby would seem to say, peculiar to the dormitories of servants, but there is not a chamber, however costly in its furniture, or ample in its dimensions, though occupied by the most cleanly and fastidious, that will not exhibit it, *if unventilated.*

Physicians have the most frequent opportunities of observing this fact, in its universality, their duty calling them continually into these apartments, and the contrast between the internal and external atmosphere, from one to the other of which they make so many transitions, being very striking. Nevertheless it may be safely said that there is not a chamber in any well-built modern house in which the accumulation of the effluvia which give rise to this peculiar odor, might not be totally prevented at the cost of a few shillings, and a little attention; and equally certain is it, that the inattention of the members of the enlightened profession of medicine to the prevalence of this evil, and its easy removal, is anything but creditable to them. The simple remedy which will be pointed out in the concluding chapter, if generally adopted would save many a doctor's visit, and dose of medicine.

The contagious viri of small-pox, measles, scarlet fever, and all others of that class, are also admitted to be communicated through the intermedium of the atmosphere, and actually inhaled by the lungs, and absorbed into the circulation. The chances of infection are, therefore, in proportion to the amount of the virus contained in the air inhaled. If the poison is allowed to concentrate, it will be obviously more dangerous than when diluted with fresh air. If, then, a person enters the chamber of a patient, sick with typhus fever, his danger will diminish in proportion to the means used to ventilate the apartment, and if this has not been attended to, he would be much safer in a well-ventilated ward of a hospital where there is a score of patients.

These destructive maladies are by no means confined to the places that have been alluded to. On the banks of the Tigris, Indus, Ganges, Niger, Amazon, in fact in all the torrid regions of the earth, and especially when cleanliness, drainage, and ventilation, have been neglected, they make their devastations; and in many of those places the probabilities of human life are alarmingly on the decrease. Many places on our own continent have become "graves for foreigners;" and the acclimated and native inhabitants, though they seem to be comparatively exempt, are taken, as it were, by stolen marches, and their fate is scarcely less sure, though it perhaps may approach with slower pace. The origin of these miasmata, the laws which govern them, and the particular diseases they engender, are still subjects of considerable controversy, and of course somewhat involved in obscurity.

This is not strange, but it is very remarkable that their *effects* are neither fully understood, nor thoroughly avoided. If this position required proof, we have only to turn to the few means that have been resorted to, to avert those effects. For example, when the plague visits Bagdad, Smyrna, or Constantinople, or when malaria visits Rome, or yellow fever New Orleans, or Portobello, those who are fortunate enough to survive, or are not openly attacked by the malady, *only* congratulate themselves on their *escape*, but never attempt to avert its return. But that *escape* is, to the most superficial observer, a serious delusion. The pallor of countenance, the languor of the corporeal, and the imbecility of the mental functions, the cadaverous aspect and premature decrepitude, are infallible indications that the poison has been imbibed, and is still lurking deeply in the circulating current, has distributed itself to every organ, physical and intellectual, and is slowly, but surely, preying upon the stamina of life, and sapping the foundations of both body and mind.

It would be almost absurd to suppose that the constant inhalation of vitiated air, should be confined to the mere generation and extension of fever. The aerial poison, when acting with less intensity, is still sufficient to affect the general health, less or more, and call into action the latent germs of other diseases. The observations of Dr. Southwood Smith on this point are so relevant, and consistent with facts daily occurring, that they must not be omitted.

" I particularize fever" (says Dr. Smith to the commissioners),* " because fever is the most obvious and the most rapidly fatal, of the diseases arising from the neglect of sewerage, ventilation, and cleanliness; but it would be a very inadequate view of the pernicious agency of the poison unceasingly generated in these filthy and neglected districts, to restrict it to the disease the most obviously produced by it. Its indirect action is highly noxious, though the evil is not so manifest. It is a matter of constant observation, that even when not present in sufficient intensity to produce fever, by disturbing the function of some organ or some set of organs, and thereby weakening the general system, this poison acts as a powerful predisposing cause, of some of the most common and fatal maladies to which the human body is subject. For example, the deaths occasioned in this coun-

* Vide " First Report of the Commissioners for inquiring into the State of large Towns and Populous Districts," p. 10.

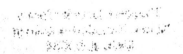

try by diseases of the digestive organs,* by inflammation of the air passages and lungs, and by consumption, form by far the largest proportion of the annual mortality. Now no one who lives long in or near a malarial district, is ever, for a single hour, free from some disease of the digestive organs. But disordered states of the digestive organs not only constitute in themselves highly painful and even fatal maladies, but they lay the foundations of several other mortal diseases. By a disordered state of the digestive organs for example, the body is often so much enfeebled that it is wholly incapable of resisting the frequent and sudden changes of temperature to which this climate is subject; the consequence is, that the person thus enfeebled, perishes by inflammation set up in some vital organ, and more especially in the air-passages and lungs; or by consumption, the consequence of that inflammation; so that to the total number of deaths, that take place, annually, from fever, in its different forms, must be added those caused by the indirect operation of the same poison that produces fever. Even when they (the causes above referred to) do not produce acute diseases, and at once lay the individual aside, they produce diseases of the nutritive system, and thus injure the constitution, diminish its power of resisting the numerous causes of disease to which the body is commonly exposed, and so enfeeble it, that the individual is very much incapacitated from labor. The gradual deterioration of health, caused by badly-ventilated dwellings, and uncleanliness, " is universally and strikingly indicated in two ways. First, by the incapacity of the mothers to attend to their children; and secondly, by the bad health of the children, and their great mortality. It has been already shown, by the experience of the fever hospital,

* Probably even more deaths proceed from diseases of the digestive organs in America than in England.

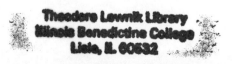

that the mothers are more susceptible of fever than the husbands, but when not laboring under any acute disease, the mothers are often so enfeebled as to be unable to attend properly to their domestic duties ; so that the children are not taken due care of, while the sickness of the children becomes an enormous tax on the time and wages of the parents. In consequence of the disease and weakness generated by the condition in which they live, the ability of the laboring classes to support themselves is very much diminished, and in very many instances, this has the effect of throwing them on parish relief. The consequent burden on private individuals and public in‧stitutions, is the least part of the evil. The great evil of this state of things, is its tendency to break down the spirit of independence, and to reduce large classes of the people to the degradation and wretchedness of depending for their support on charity, and not on their own industry."

But the deleterious effects of atmospheric poisons do not stop here, and it would be happy for the human race if those effects were only inflicted on the physical constitution ; unfortunately, their ravages extend to the mental faculties also. On this subject, the writer just quoted says : " There is evidence that as they have not the bodily vigor, and the industrious habits of a healthy and independent peasantry, so they have not the intelligence and spirit proper to such a race. One of the most melancholy proofs of this is in the quiet and unresisting manner in which they succumb to the wretchedness of their lot. They make no effort to get into happier circumstances ; their dulness and apathy indicate an equal degree of mental as of physical paralysis, and this has struck other observers, who have had opportunities of becoming acquainted with the real state of these people. In the poor law commissioner's report on the sanatory

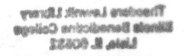

condition of the laboring population, there is the following statement, which impressed my mind the more because it recalled to my recollection, vividly, similar cases witnessed by myself. 'In the year 1836,' says one of the medical officers of the West Darby Union, 'I attended a family of thirteen — twelve of whom had typhus fever, without a bed, in the *cellar*, without straw or timber-shavings — frequent substitutes. They lay on the floor, and so crowded that I could scarcely pass between them. In another house, I attended fourteen patients — there were only two beds in the house. All the patients lay on the boards, and during their illness never had their clothes off. I met with many cases, in similar conditions, yet amidst the greatest destitution and want of domestic comfort, *I never heard, during the course of twelve years' practice, a complaint of inconvenient accommodation.*' Now this want of complaint, under such circumstances, appears to me to constitute a very melancholy part of this condition. It shows that physical wretchedness has done its worst on the human sufferer, for it has destroyed his mind. The wretchedness being greater than humanity can bear, annihilates the mental faculties — the faculties distinctive of the human being. There is a kind of satisfaction in the thought, for it sets a limit to the capacity of suffering, which would otherwise be without bound."

9

CHAPTER IX.

CONSUMPTION.—Number of Deaths by it in Great Britain and the United States.—Statement of Dr. Guy.—Its relative Prevalence among Professional Men, Tradesmen, and Artisans.—Experience of a London Tradesman.—Fresh Air retards its Development when Hereditary.—Its relative Prevalence among Males and Females in Town and Country.—Table.—Workshops.—Inhalation of Dust, Fumes, metallic Particles, &c.—SCROFULA.—Tubercles.—Food not Nutritive unless Aerated.—Opinion of M. Baudelocque of the Causes of Scrofula.—Long-continued Respiration of Foul Air not necessary to Produce it.—Shepherds.—Sleeping with the Head Covered.—Illustration.—Village of Oresmeaux.—Opinion of Sir James Clark.—Scrofula Producible in a healthy Infant.—Prevalent among Rabbits, Monkeys, Cows, Horses.—Curious Medical Practice in Scotland.—Physical Education.—Scrofula in the Norwood School; its cause and Cure.—Relation of Animal Composition and the Development of Respiratory Apparatus.—Constructions of the Chest.—Leaning against Desks.—*Tight-Lacing;* its Effects.—Coroner's Verdict in such Cases.

NEXT *to those maladies which are the more obvious products of the respiration of vitiated air, and which have been called pestilential, or contagious, may perhaps be classed those of the respiratory organs themselves.* These are too numerous to be mentioned in detail, and may all be directly produced by breathing air insufficient in quantity, bad in quality, or of improper temperature. *Consumption* has been looked upon, in all ages, as one of the most formidable diseases, and though it proceeds from a variety of causes, none operate more effectively in its production than sedentary occupations, changes of the atmospheric temperature, unprovided against by proper means, and living in houses or working in manufactories, or coal-pits, &c., where ventilation has not been attended to. Hence, in England, where these causes are in constant operation, and where pit coal is burned to a great extent, consumption is particularly prevalent. In the days of Arbuthnot, consumption made up one tenth of the bills of mortality in the city of London, an estimate which has been lately increased to one fourth. It is also probable that as many as 100,000 die of consumption, in the British isles, in one year. Dr. Alcott supposes himself safe in stating the annual mortality from consumption, of the United States, at 50,000, or 1,000,000 every twenty years. In fine, consumption is found to prevail to the greatest extent in crowded cities, where the air is confined or impregnated with noxious matters, and this fact sufficiently proves of itself, that impure air is at least one of the most prevalent causes of consumption. Dr. Guy, in his examination on this point, before the commissioners, affirms, " This [deficient ventilation] I believe to be more fatal than all other causes put together." He briefly states the result of his inquiries respecting the cause of consumption, with a view to prove its origin, from impure and confined air, thus : —

" 1st. Consumption is relatively more frequent in persons working in doors, than those employed out of doors

" 2d. In those employed within doors, it is most frequent in men using little exertion.

" 3d. It makes its attacks earlier where it is of most frequent occurrence.

" 4th. It is very common in the intemperate, and in those exposed to the inhalation of dust.

" 5th. It is more frequent in men than women, at least in the metropolis (London)."

It also appears from Dr. Guy's evidence, that of the three classes, of *gentlemen* (including professional men), *tradesmen* (storekeepers), and *artisans*, including laborers of every class, the cases of consumption stand as the numbers, 16, 28, and 30. From this it follows that the

tradesmen of London (and they are pretty similarly circumstanced in New York and the other great cities of
this country), are nearly twice as liable to consumption as
the gentry.   This great mortality Dr. Guy mainly attributes to the confinement during so many hours of every
day, in ill-ventilated shops.   In large cities, tradesmen
and shopmen suffer occasionally from the way in which
they are lodged or housed.   They give up to their business all the space they can command, and let the upper
part of their houses to lodgers, living themselves in small
back rooms, connected with their stores, which rooms are
not larger or better ventilated than those of the poor.
This leads to much sickness among them.   " It is," continues Dr. Guy, " only within a few days, that a London
tradesman gave me this account of himself.—He had
been originally a workman, and having saved a little
money, opened a small shop in a back street.   For some
years he slept in a small close back room, behind his shop;
and during the whole time was subject to frequent attacks
of cold, with affection of the chest.   These attacks were
often so severe as to require medical advice and attend-
ance, for weeks together.   He has since moved into an
open airy situation, with ample accommodation for himself and family, and he is not only very rarely subject to
colds, but these when they do occur, are readily cured,
by the most simple means.   He states that he saves in
this way a large sum, previously expended on medicine."
Had the tradesman in this case persisted in his former
way of living and sleeping, consumption, in its incurable
form, would in all probability have been the result.

It has been observed that where there is a predisposition to consumption, pure air retards the progress of
the disease, and prevents its development until late in life,
and *vice versa*.   Hawkers and carriers who stand, sit, or
journey from place to place, exposed to the inclemency,

and all the vicissitudes of the weather, are known to be not only less subject to consumption, but if they die of it, die later than those who work indoors, and are protected from the weather. Except imperfect ventilation be assumed as the cause of the greater frequency of consumption, and its more rapid termination, among indoor laborers, than among those engaged in the open air, we are unable to account for this well-ascertained fact. All circumstances but the one specified, are in favor of the former class. Their wages are higher, and consequently their food, clothing, lodging, &c., are of better quality, and it is probable they are somewhat less addicted to intemperance, yet all these advantages do not compensate for the want of pure air. The greater mortality of males, compared with that of females, Dr. Guy attributes to the fact that the latter are not so much employed in working in companies together, but frequently work in their own rooms. Though this is true with regard to London, the result is just the contrary in manufacturing districts and towns where many females are employed. Their more delicate constitutions are not so able to withstand the gradual deterioration of the pulmonary apparatus, produced by breathing air that has passed through many lungs, and lost the great bulk of its vivifying principle, before it arrives at theirs, and they of course contract consumption, and sink under it more readily than the other sex, whose lungs and constitution are more robust. Milliners, dressmakers, tailors, shoemakers, pressmen, and compositors, apart from the injurious effects of the bent positions of their bodies, and the consequent diminished capacities of their chests, are particularly exposed to the influence of repeatedly-inhaled and otherwise vitiated air. The high rents of large rooms in large cities, demand economy of space, and therefore the employers are disposed to huddle together the workers, or

9*

as the London tailors express it, set them "*knee to knee and elbow to elbow.*" The employers are not solely to be blamed ; we must suppose the workers to be instrumental in lowering the standard of their own health and morality, and knowingly or unwittingly inflicting upon themselves a lingering but generally certain self-destruction, while their heartless masters or mistresses are all but guilty of the slow and insidious murder of a class of their fellow-creatures, which comprises some of the most useful members of the community. Indeed, these classes are seldom without catarrh, headache, rheumatism, pains in the chest, debility, indigestion, or spitting of blood, which usually pave the way for incurable consumption, and in a short time, by undermining the constitution, realize the picture that has been just drawn. As a confirmation of the injurious effects attributed to impure air, Dr. Guy gives the following table, founded upon a careful inquiry into the condition of some letter-press printers, as to health, and an accurate measurement of the rooms in which they were employed : —

					Per centage proportion.			
	Spitting of Blood.	Ca-tarrh	Other Diseases.	Total	Spitting of Blood.	Ca-tarrh.	Other Diseases.	Total.
104 men having less than 500 cubic feet of air to breathe,	13	13	18	44	12·50	12 5	17·31	42·31
115 men with from 500 to 600 cubic ft. of air to breathe,	5	4	23	32	4·35	3·48	20 00	27 82
101 men with more than 600 cubic feet of air to breathe,	4	2	18	24	3·96	1·98	17·82	23·76

So far from limiting the influence of vitiated air to the production of consumption, or even confining the consequences of that influence to the body, Dr. Guy further states, "I consider the heated and impure atmosphere of

workshops, and a similarly unwholesome state of the
dwellings of the poor, as the cause of a large number of
diseases—of scrofulous diseases in childhood, of inflammation of the lungs, of the febrile affections, to which the
children of the poor are so subject, and of those chronic
disorders of the bowels, which are so apt to terminate in
mesenteric disease.—A great proportion of the deaths of
children entered in the reports of the registrar-general, as
consumption, are of this nature, and chiefly due to this
cause. In adults the effect of the depressing atmosphere
of places of work, such as those described, extends much
beyond the production of pulmonary consumption. Both
the mind and the body are injured; the one is in a state
to be excited by slight causes, and the other to require,
or to seem to require, the aid of intoxicating liquors. Each
ministers to the other's weakness, and each reacts upon
the other. I believe that as a general rule men who
work out of doors drink more than those employed within doors; they have more temptations; they are more
in the way of it. But I believe that the unwholesome
state of places of work, by the depressing effect it produces, is a great cause of intemperance. It can scarcely be otherwise."—Dr. Guy sums up his evidence in the
following terms: "There is no sufficient reason for considering consumption as an English disease. A certain
amount of consumption, probably about one in seven of
all deaths above fifteen years of age, which is nearly the
proportion occurring in the higher orders, and in the
most healthy professions, may be considered as inevitable; but all beyond that proportion admits of prevention.
The annual waste of adult-life from pulmonary consumption alone, may be safely stated at upward of five thousand, and this estimate is probably much below the truth.
The chief cause of this great mortality is the defective ventilation of houses, shops, and places of work. Next to this,

in point of importance, is the inhalation of dust, metallic particles, and irritating fumes. One cause, over which the poor themselves can exercise control, is the abuse of spirituous liquors, a very fruitful source of consumption. I will venture to add my own strong conviction, that the sacrifice of so large a number of grown-up men and women, has the indirect effect of decreasing the population, of substituting young and helpless children, for adults capable of earning their own subsistence, and of contributing to the wealth and greatness of their country; that this waste of adult-life is, in every sense and view of the matter, a great calamity, and very bad economy, and to the extent to which its causes are generally understood by individuals, or by the public, a great and cruel injustice."

Consumption is very often, if not always, a SYMPTOM *of a disease which assumes different forms, and which is known by the generic term* SCROFULA. Many have attempted to draw a distinction between the two but not succesfully.   S. Cooper,* Alison, and many of the best authorities recognise the full identity of these diseases. Scrofula usually shows itself in suppurating tumors, in various parts of the body, internally and externally, enlargement of the glands of the neck, and mesentery, and often in the development of small bodies in the substance of the lungs, and other parts, named *tubercles.* These tubercles are of various forms, colors, and consistence, and generally of a pale yellowish color, and seldom exceeding the size of a small pea. As to their origin and chemical composition, little certain is known, though these points have been made subjects of the most careful investigation. From the very discrepant analyses that have been made from time to time, to ascertain their elements, it may be inferred that their chemical constituents are variable in

* Vide Cooper's Surgical Dictionary, article Scrofula.

different subjects. They are developed in almost every tissue of the body, especially in the lungs, in which case the disease is called *pulmonary consumption* or *tubercular phthisis*. They are also frequently found in the liver, the reason of which will be attempted to be explained. The circumstance of their being found in large numbers in the lungs, even when the other structures are comparatively exempt, is of itself strong presumptive evidence that their original formation is intimately connected with the function of respiration, though it does not *prove* that an obstruction in that function is the proximate cause of their growth. The ablest modern physiologists contend that tubercles are morbid products, resulting from abortive attempts at organization. This accident results from various causes affecting the *nutritive process*, or that process which prepares the blood, in sufficient quantity and quality, for the formation of living structures.

As three principal causes have been alleged, viz.: hereditary predisposition, insufficient or unwholesome food, and an insufficient supply of pure air, the question for our immediate purpose naturally resolves itself into the inquiry, which of these causes has been observed to operate most strongly in producing consumption, scrofula, or other disease, indicated more or less by the presence of tubercles? It is to be hoped the opinions about to be adduced will constitute a satisfactory answer.

It is however necessary here to explain, that a universality of cause producing scrofula, to the exclusion of all others, is not contended for. An attempt will only be made to bring forward satisfactory evidence, to show that deficient aeration of the blood is the *principal cause*, and that hereditary tendency, bad diet, depressing passions, too late, too early, or in-and-in marriages, sedentary occupations, want of exercise, deficient clothing, bad water, &c., which have been separately and collectively alleged by writers, are only secondary and auxiliary in their operation.

In the first place, there is strong reason to believe that the blood corpuscles are mainly affected in the function of respiration, and it is possible to show, by both philosophical principles and established facts, that the want of due arterialization of the blood, by a sufficiently oxygenated air, is essentially connected with the state of the blood which exists in this disease. Dr. Carpenter, one of the most successful pathologists of the present time, after enumerating the various effects of insufficiency of air, or suspension of the aerating process, says : "Again the due elaboration of the *fibrin* of the blood, is undoubtedly prevented by an habitually deficient respiration, and various diseases which result from the imperfect performance of this elaboration, consequently manifest themselves. The *scrofulous* diathesis is thus frequently connected with an unusually small capacity of the chest. If there be an imperfect elaboration of the nutrient materials, as happens in the tuberculous diathesis, its effects are peculiarly liable to manifest themselves at this period [youth] when the demand for nutritive matter is greatly augmented by the activity of the muscular system."

Now it is not disputed, that matter, carried from the digestive organs, and thrown into the circulation, can not be perfectly nutritive, unless it be perfectly aerated or oxygenated. This fact is fully established. A very small quantity of food, even when it is to a certain extent unwholesome, may possibly be assimilated, and with a due supply of air to ventilate it when it arrives at the lungs, may become highly nutritive ; but the largest conceivable quantity of what is called nutritious food, taken into the stomach, and there digested, can never be elaborated into nutritive blood, without a due supply of air to arterialize it.

M. Baudelocque, a celebrated French writer, has made the causes of this disease a subject of the most careful investigation, and as his opinions have been pretty generally adopted by the best physicans in Europe and America, and are in accordance with our own experience, it will perhaps be necessary to make a few quotations from his treatise, "Observations sur les Maladies Scrofuleuse."

" Invariably it will be found, on examination, that a truly *scrofulous* disease is caused by a vitiated air, and *it is not always necessary that there should have been a prolonged stay in such an atmosphere.* Often a few hours each day is sufficient, and it is thus they may live in the most healthy country, pass the greater part of the day in the open air, and yet become scrofulous because of sleeping in a confined place, where the air has not been renewed. This is the case with many shepherds. It is usual to attribute scrofula, in their case, to exposure to storms and atmospheric changes, and to humidity. But attention has not been paid to the circumstance, that they pass the night in a confined hut, which they transport from place to place, and which guaranties them against humidity : this hut has only a small door, which is closed when they enter, and remains closed also during the day : six or eight hours passed daily in a vitiated air, and which no draught ever removes, is the true cause of their disease. I have spoken of the bad habit of sleeping with the head under the clothes, and the insalubrity of the *classes* where a number of children are assembled together. The repetition of these circumstances is often sufficient cause of scrofula, although they may last but for a few hours a day." He supports this view by the following striking instance : " At three leagues from Amiens lies the village of Oresmeaux ; it is situated in a vast plain, open on every side, and elevated more than a hundred feet above the neighboring valleys. About sixty years ago most of the houses were built of clay, and had no windows; they were lighted by one or two panes of glass fixed in the wall; none of the floors, sometimes many feet below the level of the street, were paved. The ceilings were low, the greater part of the inhabitants were engaged in weaving. A few holes in the wall, and which were closed at will by means of a plank, scarcely permitted the light and air to penetrate into the workshop. Humidity was thought necessary to keep the threads fresh. Nearly all the inhabitants were seized with scrofula, and many families continually ravaged by that malady became extinct,—their last members as they write me, died *rotten with scrofula.* A fire destroyed nearly one third of the village: the houses were rebuilt in a more salubrious manner, and by degrees scrofula became less common and disappeared from that part. Twenty years later another third of the village was consumed; the same amelioration in building with a like effect, as to scrofula. The disease is now confined to the inhabitants of the older houses which retain the same causes of insalubrity."

It is unnecessary to cross the Atlantic to see the depopulating effect of damp and underground residences. New York has enough cellar-residents to make another Oresmeaux, and their mortality must also be nearly if not quite equal.

In speaking of the hereditary descent of the disease, Baudelocque admits that scrofula may be propagated from parents to their offspring, but adduces numerous examples that tend to diminish very much the importance generally attached to hereditary constitution as a cause of the disease, and which prove that it is possible to destroy the predisposition, and to avoid the malady, by simply respiring pure air. He further asserts that " when the parents have ceased to be scrofulous, they can only transmit to their children a predisposition to the disease, of which they are cured. To develop this disease, it is necessary that the children find themselves placed under the atmospheric condition of which I have spoken; that they habitually respire an air whose principal constituents are altered. In consequence of their predisposition to scrofula, it is true it will show itself more readily in their case, than in that of other children exposed to the same cause, but the action of a vitiated air is always necessary to the development of the disease; to withdraw from the one is to avoid the other, whatever may be the hereditary disposition. Finally, M. Baudelocque affirms, that the repeated respiration of the same atmosphere is a primary and efficient cause of scrofula, and that " if there be entirely pure air, there may be bad food, bad clothing, and want of personal cleanliness, but that scrofulous disease can not exist," and supports this assertion by numerous cases and incontrovertible facts. Dr. Duncan, who has also devoted very great attention to the causes of scrofula, corroborates the opinions of M. Baudelocque in these terms : " It seems natural to expect that the organs with which the foreign gaseous ingredients of the atmosphere come more immediately into contact, and whose blood-vessels they must enter on their passage into the system, should feel in a distinctive manner, their noxious influence, and this *a-priori* expectation is strengthened by the observation, in both man and animals, as well as by experiment on the latter. It has been observed that when individuals breathe habitually impure air, and are exposed to the other debilitating causes which must always influence more or less the inhabitants of dark, filthy, and ill-ventilated dwellings, scrofula — and consumption as one of its forms — are very apt to be engendered, even when the hereditary predisposition to the disease may be

10

absent." Professor Alison, one of the highest authorities on this subject, remarks: " It is hardly possible to observe separately, the effect on the animal economy of deficiency of exercise, and deficiency of fresh air, these two causes being very generally applied together, and often in connexion with imperfect nourishment. But it is perfectly ascertained, on an extensive scale, in regard to the inhabitants of large and crowded cities, as compared with the rural population of the same climate—first, that their mortality is very much greater, especially in early life, and the probability of life very much less ; and, secondly, that of this great early mortality in large towns, a very large proportion is caused by scrofulous disease. And from these two facts, it evidently follows that deficiency of fresh air, and of exercise, are among the most powerful and the most important, because often the most remediable, of the causes from which the scrofulous diathesis arises."

Sir J. Clark, who has written the best monograph on consumption in our language, regards the respiration of a deteriorated atmosphere, as one of the most powerful causes of tuberculous cachexia, that is, the constitutional affection which precedes the appearance of consumption. He says: " If an infant born in perfect health, and of the healthiest parents, be kept in close rooms, in which free ventilation and cleanliness are neglected, a few months will often suffice to induce tuberculous cachexia."— "There can be no doubt," he adds, " that the habitual respiration of the air of ill-ventilated and gloomy alleys in large towns, is a powerful means of augmenting the hereditary disposition to scrofula, and even of inducing such a disposition *de novo*. Children reared in the workhouses of this country, and in similar establishments abroad, almost all become scrofulous, and this more, we believe, from the confined impure atmosphere in which they live, and the want of active exercise, than from defective nourishment." The same distinguished physician has actually succeeded in inducing consumption in rabbits, by confining them in cold, damp, dark, close situations, and supplying them with innutritious food. Monkeys present the same phenomenon in this country, where they are often crowded together during the winter in a confined and heated atmosphere, and where true tubercular consumption commits more extensive ravages among them, than it does among the human race.

It is believed also that this malady is very prevalent among cows which supply milk to the inhabitants of some large towns, where they are immured during part of every year, in close dairies, and which being too small for the number of animals they contain, soon become filled with heated, vitiated air, for the removal of which no provision has been made! Can those persons who use the milk of such cows escape disease? It is to be feared that a negative conclusion can not be escaped. Indeed, to suppose that the material of the milk could pass into, and through, four stomachs, be absorbed into the chyliferous ducts, and thence thrown into the circulation, perform many rounds in the blood-vessels, be elaborated into milk by a complicated process in the glandular apparatus, and after it has come in contact with diseased tissues in every step of its progress, possibly remain a considerable time in the body of the animal, and yet not be tainted with morbific qualities, would be utterly repugnant to reason and experience.

It is also more than probable, that horses kept in ill-ventilated stables are often attacked with contagious diseases, which are readily communicated to the human species; and it is not very unusual to hear of hostlers and others falling a prey to the disease called *glanders*, which is commonly supposed to be a morbid secretion from the mucous membrane lining the air passages of the nose, the result of a scrofulous condition of that tissue, and which is only a symptom of an extensive and latent tuberculous disease. In these cases the culpable disregard of a proper supply of pure air to these poor animals, on the part of their keepers, is obviously the cause of the destruction of both.

As an illustration of some of the unaccountable infatuations under which the comparatively well-informed labor, with regard to the purity of air, it may be mentioned that in some parts of Scotland, even at the present day, when a person begins to complain of consumption, he is very gravely advised by his friends, or some old woman, who is often the "*family doctor*," to live for a certain number of days in the cowhouse ! To do justice, however, to that enlightened nation, it must be acknowledged that this *practice* is generally ridiculed, and fast falling into the disrepute it so well merits.*

Too much credit can scarcely be given to those few philanthropists, who have begun to interest themselves in, or rather revive, the cause of physical education. This will be admitted, when it is recollected that of late volumes above volumes have been written, on the best methods of " Mental Education," moral and intellectual training, &c., and a very unamiable controversial temper has occasionally been indulged in, by the advocates of the respective systems—so different are their theories. But they all seem to be agreed on one point: that physical training is, at best, a merely secondary and unimportant consideration. They teach the children a whole encyclopedia of knowledge, classic, and modern. They make the schools, as it were, forcing beds for the growth of intellect ; without seeming to reflect, that it is at the expense of the constitutions of their pupils. They ad-

* Vide Dr. Andrews' Dictionary of Domestic Medicine.

mire the intellectual precocity of a child, without making allowance for that waste of physical, and consequently mental energy, which never can be restored, and which will be found wanting when most required. The best wish, and the most rational one, that can present itself to the human mind is contained in the proverb "*mens sana in corpore sano;*" yet this principle, clear though it be, is in these schools hardly ever inculcated, and very generally disregarded. Instances might be multiplied without number, to justify these statements, but one connected with the subject, at present under discussion, will perhaps suffice. In 1832, at Norwood school, in England, where there were six hundred pupils, scrofula broke out, extensively, among the children, and carried off great numbers. This was at once ascribed to bad and insufficient food. Dr. Arnott was, however, employed to investigate the matter, and immediately decided that the food was "*most abundant and good,*" assigning "*defective ventilation, and consequent atmospheric impurity,*" as the true cause. Ventilation was accordingly applied by his direction; the scrofula soon disappeared, and eleven hundred children are now maintained, in good health, where the six hundred, before a proper system of ventilation was adopted, were scrofulous and sickly.*

In all classes of animals there is found a certain relation between the composition of the body and the development of the apparatus of respiration, which may account for the production of scrofula by breathing foul air. In a work on the "Lungs and their Diseases," by James Stewart, M. D., of New York, may be found the rudiments of an explanation of the mode in which scrofulous

---

* For numerous other well-authenticated instances of a similar nature, see Toynbee's Evidence before the Commissioners, 1st Report, p. 78, et seq.

10*

tubercles result from the inspiration of too little, or too foul, an air.

It is remarked that in the lowest form of animal organization, *albumen* predominates greatly over all other animalized substances. In the egg, it forms nearly the whole mass, and so in the oyster, the muscle, and other similar organizations. As animals rise in the scale of being, this substance is reduced in proportion to the whole mass of the body, growing less in the fish, still less in the reptile, and diminishing with each increase of perfection of animal powers, until the highest is attained to in the bird, the more active quadrupeds, and in man himself.

Now if we compare these different classes of beings in another particular, we find a remarkable coincidence, viz.: that in those of the lowest organization, *respiration is least active*, and as they rise in the scale, respiration becomes more and more elaborate. In other words, the greater the proportion of albumen in the animal, the less important is the function of respiration; and the less the proportion of albumen, the more complicated, more developed, and more important, is this function.

Thus in the egg, respiration is at its lowest point.* Then in the oyster, muscle, &c., there is found a more elaborate, though still an exceedingly meager, respiratory apparatus. In the more active fishes, whose bodies contain less albumen, there is a still greater elaboration of respiration, though all the air they get is found in the water they inhabit, except in a few species which have lungs, and must rise to the surface to get the necessary amount of air. The latter (whales, &c.), have still less of albumen in their composition, its place being supplied

---

* Some may think that an egg does not breathe at all. But a simple experiment will show that exposure to the air is necessary to the continuance of the life of an egg. Let the shell be covered with a thin coat of wax or even a single layer of varnish, and it will soon begin to decay.

by fat and oil. As we ascend in the examination to reptiles, &c., we find a more perfect respiration still, and less albumen, and so on upward, till we arrive at birds, and man, which have the largest proportionate breathing apparatus.

The next fact to be noticed in connexion with this subject, is, *the composition of scrofulous tubercle.* Chemical analysis shows this substance to consist almost wholly of albumen, the very substance of which those animals are formed, who possess the smallest respiration. As is stated by Dr. Stewart, " The matter contained in all scrofulous tumors, whether they are external or situated in the lungs, is precisely the same. It consists of pale, opake albumen, more or less coagulated, resembling sometimes the whey, at other times the curds, of milk. Analysis shows that the animalized part of the matter contained in these tumors *consists exclusively of albumen ;* being 98·15 parts in 100, the remainder 1·85 is nothing but salts of lime and soda."

Now, it has been shown in the preceding pages, that scrofula in human beings and other animals, is the direct result of the respiration of too little, or too impure, an atmosphere. Animal blood contains a considerable portion of albumen derived doubtless from the food consumed. A chemical combination of this fluid with the oxygen of the air, is necessary to fit it for nourishing the body properly, and *to prevent the deposite of this albumen in its nearly pure form.* If it does not combine with the oxygen of the air in sufficient quantity to change its character, *it will be deposited in the form of tubercle,* and we then have scrofula, indicated by those deposites.

Man may, therefore, be reduced from his higher and more elaborate animal condition, to a condition nearer that of animals of inferior organization, by imperfect respiration, and the consequent development in his body, of a substance of which those inferior beings are composed; a substance which is entirely natural to them, but destructive to him; a substance which they can not live without, but which he can not live with.

Exposed to the full influence of the atmosphere these albuminous animals can not live, though in their native element they appropriate to themselves some of the oxygen it contains. It may be that they die in the air, because of too much oxygen being absorbed into their systems, changing the character of the albumen of which they are principally and naturally composed; as man would die by the respiration of pure oxygen, or of an atmosphere containing more than its natural proportion of that gas.

On the other hand, man, and the other more perfect animals, must have a sufficiency of oxygen to exert a proper chemical influence upon the albumen contained naturally in their blood, otherwise, it will, if not thus changed, be deposited *as albumen alone,* and where thus deposited, it operates as a foreign substance, interrupts the natural function of the part where it is located, or excites inflammation by the irritation it produces, resulting in disorganization and death.

This view of the subject will perhaps also reasonably account for the deposition of scrofulous tubercles in those tissues where they are most frequently found, viz., in the glands and in the lungs.

The glands of the body are the principal organs of secretion; that is, the organs which separate from the blood, the different materials of which the body is composed. The lungs, as the reader has already learned, are the organs in which the blood is brought into direct contact with the air, and where the action of the oxygen of the air on the albumen of the blood is first exerted. The glands and lungs are the main points of the alteration of the blood, and therefore, on the reasoning above, they are the points at which an imperfect operation would be most likely to be first noticed,—and where, in fact, scrofulous tubercle is most abundant.

Thus there may be said to be established a uniform relation between the air and the albumen of all animal bodies.

Anything that tends to restrict the chest to unnatural limits, must necessarily diminish the volume of air inhaled, and thus there is an insufficient quantity of oxygen to vitalize the blood, even in a well-ventilated apartment, or in the open air. This is especially applicable to those persons of sedentary or studious habits, whose lungs are externally compressed by working with the body curved forward, as in the case of tailors, shoemakers, engravers, etc., and especially those who have contracted the habit of leaning forward on the table or desk on which they write. In ill-ventilated schools, where a number of circumstances combine to depress the spirits, and render the body languid, nothing is more common than to see the children lean with the whole weight of their bodies, on the desks, while they read or write; and this cause (which is very often overlooked) operates as one of the most powerful and efficient auxiliaries, in producing consumption and scrofula. Tight-lacing, or the unnatural constriction of the waists of females, has even a greater effect in impeding the healthy exercise of the function of respiration, and is of course attended with more permanent and fatal results. In this function, the diaphragm plays by far the most important part. Indeed when a rib is broken, and absolute quiescence of the walls of the chest is enjoined by the surgeon, respiration may possibly be carried on by the diaphragm alone. But when the waist is constrained into an hour-glass form, the liver, stomach, and part of the bowels, lying immediately below the diaphragm, are forced up and press against that muscle, wholly, or partially, preventing its action, and exciting in it a morbid irritability, and sometimes excessive vomiting, as is often evinced in the case of sea-sickness,* but which is pretty common among those ladies, who have adopted the pernicious custom referred to, and who "*always admire a slender waist,*" though the other sex are generally of an opposite taste!

Passing over biliary derangements, rickets, curvature of the spine, &c., as somewhat irrelevant to the present subject, it will be easy to establish a connexion between consumption, and this absurd burlesque on the creative skill of the Almighty.

It has been stated, in a previous part of this work, that respiration is produced mainly by the diaphragm, which is convex on its upper side, contracting and enlarging the cavity of the chest which produces a vacuum, into which, during the free and unrestricted action of the muscle a sufficient volume of air rushes. Now it is quite plain, that when the viscera, mentioned above, press forcibly upward, the contraction of the muscle is prevented, and the quantity of air inhaled, very much diminished. It is also as plain, that all the functions of life will become impaired, from the scanty oxygenation of the blood, dyspepsia, headache, diseases of the heart, peculiar ir-regularities of the female system, hysterics, consumption, and scrofula, will ensue, as a necessary consequence; and the pallor of countenance, emaciation of frame, and meaningless aspect, too surely indicate that inroads have been made, on both the physical and mental energies; and it will be found that hypochondriasis, that most mis-erable of all diseases, or rather class of diseases, derives

---

* Sea-sickness is by some supposed to be chiefly the result of the pressure of the lower viscera upon the diaphragm, the immediate consequence of the body being rapidly carried downward, when the more yielding parts are as it were left behind, or make a sudden rush upward.

its origin oftener from the abuse of the respiratory function, than any other cause.

The assertion may be safely hazarded, that thousands of deaths have occurred, among females, which, had they been made subjects of investigation before a coroner's jury, would have truly warranted the verdict of *self-murder*. Such would be the verdict in an ordinary case of hanging, between which and *suffocation by the waist* it is impossible to draw any further distinction, than that the constriction is applied to different parts of the body, and that, in one case, the operation is more lingering, and not so rapidly fatal, as it is in the other. It is, however, a source of consolation to those interested in the progress of civilization, and the amelioration of public health, that "*hour-glass waists*" as they have been very appropriately termed, are fast giving place to true taste, and will shortly, instead of captivating the eye, be only looked upon with pity or disgust; exciting in those they are intended to please, as compassionate a smile as could be bestowed upon the fashionable follies of the reign of Queen Elizabeth, when the toes of the shoes were tied up to the knees, to prevent them from tripping the wearers. Thus may they become matter of history, and no longer contribute their share, in the degeneration of the human race, by entailing a multitude of diseases, on a miserable, but irresponsible offspring.

CHAPTER X.

Further Considerations of the Ultimate Objects of Respiration.—Relations of the Liver and Lungs — Strasburg Pies.—Influence of checked Perspiration.—Aqueous Vapor of Respiration.—*Dysentery*, occurring in Prisons.—Milbank Penitentiary.—Sing-Sing.—Auburn.—Law of " Sympathetic Association."—Action of Impure Air on the Eye.—Smoking and Drinking—Evidence of Dr. Toynbee.—Diseases of the Ear.—Effects of Bad Air on Surgical Operations.—Hospital Gangrene.—Rights and Duties of Surgeons.

Reverting to the ultimate objects of respiration, it is obvious, from their very nature, that various diseases, and even death, may be often produced, by any cause tending to obstruct the healthy operation of the function. The depurating process effected on the blood, by the absorption of oxygen, and the liberation of carbon, is *necessary to prevent the decomposition of that fluid,* and eventually of all the tissues of the body. Indeed, the abstraction of carbon from the blood, is so indispensably necessary, that when suspended, all the processes of organic life, as nutrition, secretion, formation of the tissues, reproduction, &c., together with the muscular and nervous energy, cease finally and for ever, and spontaneous decomposition of the whole body takes place. This tendency to spontaneous decomposition is, therefore, impending every moment, and can only be avoided by the prompt and efficient removal of the carbonaceous particles from the blood, which, if allowed to accumulate, would, in proportion to their amount, gradually or speedily induce decomposition, and complete disorganization. For example, in the inflammatory stage of fever, the constitution makes extraordinary efforts to rid itself of carbon, but the low typhoid stage is always associated with diminished evolution of this substance, and it gradually decreases as death approaches. After death, animals give out carbon in very large quantities, which combines with the oxygen of the air, and forms carbonic acid, an invariable result of the decomposition of all animal matter. On these principles, it is easy and reasonable to account for the origin of a great number of diseases, especially that bad habit of body to which we have already adverted as comprising a whole catalogue of ailments, usually described under the general term — *scrofula.*

But the process of respiration, does not even stop here. It not only removes useless and pernicious carbon, and prepares and preserves in a state of purity, a fluid capable of affording to all the parts of the body the materials necessary to maintain their vital endowments, but is also employed to separate any injurious matter accidentally received into, or retained in, the system, which is a circumstance of more frequent occurrence than is commonly suspected. In this way, healthy and unimpeded respiration will often purify the blood from miasmata, thus preventing the development of fever, or other contagious or pestilential diseases; — and conversely, when no regard is paid to fresh air, and a vitiated atmosphere is inhaled, these diseases are very often, as it were, invited and fostered, in their incubation, to a fatal maturity. Dr. Carpenter remarks that " there can be little doubt that the respiratory function is also an important means of purifying the blood from various deleterious matters either introduced from without (such as narcotic poisons), or generated within the body (such as the poison of fever").*

It must here be observed that Dr. C. holds (and with

* Vide El. Physiology, Am. ed., p. 431.

11

good reason) that a small amount of poisonous matter, introduced from without, in the form of contagion, or miasm, may lead, by a process resembling fermentation, to the production of a large quantity of similar noxious substances in the animal fluids. Thus a copious supply of pure air will very often, of itself, eliminate morbid matter through the lungs, which, if allowed to remain, would have produced fatal results.

It has been noticed by physiologists that the liver and respiratory organs are developed in an inverse proportion to one another, in the different classes of animals — the liver being largest, where the respiration is most feeble, and vice versa. Now this would at once lead us to suspect that there were intimate relations existing between the functions of the lungs and liver, and that consequently a derangement in one, would be followed by disease in the other. Accordingly we find, that the functional activity of the liver is greater as the amount of respiration is less ; and that the carbon, which is eliminated by the lungs, when *their* activity is the greatest, is thrown upon the *liver* for separation from the blood when the respiration is feeble. But the liver soon becomes incapable of performing this vicarious office, imposed so oppressively upon it, and becomes itself exhausted and diseased. This is more especially the case in warm climates, or under the influence of high temperature : as under these circumstances the carbonic acid is tardy in its escape from the lungs, and therefore the liver is peculiarly liable to derangement, if extraordinary attention be not paid to the air inhaled.

The effects of diminished respiration in producing diseased conditions of the liver is very strikingly exemplified, in the production of the celebrated Strasburg pies. These consist chiefly of the livers of geese — the poor animals being closely confined, for a length of time, in a high temperature, so that the respiration is reduced to its minimum, by the combined effects of warmth and muscular inaction. They are, moreover, crammed with the most nutritive food, and the consequence is, that the liver is totally unable to separate the superabundant fatty particles from the blood, which soon engorge its cells, and morbidly enlarge its dimensions. No humane person could, however, relish these pies, if conscious of the refinement in cruelty practised in their preparation. A similar diseased condition of the liver exhibits itself in man, as the result of obstructed aeration of the blood, and the engorgement of the liver, consequent on that obstruction. This accounts for much of the "liver complaint," and "fatty degeneration of the liver" of warm and temperate climates, and so often observed in the last stages of pulmonary consumption.

It is natural to pause here, and reflect for a moment what wonders of this character would be revealed to the world, if a peep could be obtained at the biliary organs (*in situ*) of many who are every day walking the streets of some of our dusty, crowded, and ill-ventilated American cities, and especially those of the fair sex, whose livers are not only congested by the ordinary want of fresh air, but also compressed, externally, with a zeal and industry that are morally due to the preservation of life, instead of being devoted to its destruction.

Could the above supposition be verified, it is also not unlikely that the principal materials of *patés*, very analogous to their prototypes at Strasburg, would present themselves in endless variety.

Under the head of diseases attributable to impure or insufficient air, may be classed those complaints which arise from a too-suddenly checked perspiration. It has been already shown that fever may possibly arise from the emanations of the sensible perspiration, in a putrid state; but the too sudden occlusion of the pores of the exhalents of the skin, is equally as fertile a source of disease. Indeed there should not, if possible, be any such thing as *sensible* perspiration. It is always a necessary evil—may be looked upon as a morbid product—and always attended by more or less constitutional derangement. No doubt, in profuse perspiration, the cutaneous capillaries (or small hairlike tubes which emit the sweat) which were congested, relieve the system by giving vent to the fluid, but when the elimination of that fluid is suddenly suspended, and the minute mouths of the exhalent vessels occluded by a rapid transition from a warm to a cold air, the internal organs, and especially the mucous membranes, are congested by a recession of the liquor, that ought to have passed through the skin by *insensible* perspiration. Irritation always follows this congestion, and hence after over-crowding in ill-ventilated churches, assemblies, schools, &c., sudden contact with the cold air very often checks the pulmonary and cutaneous transudation, and the determination of blood to the mucous membranes of the internal organs, co-operating with the already depressed state of the general system produced by the inhalation of carbonic acid, lays the foundation of numerous pulmonary diseases, such as croup, thrush, pneumonia, pleurisy, chronic catarrhs, asthmas, &c., that render miserable, and abridge human life. Some of the diseases just specified, are also favored in their development, by the retention of the *aqueous vapor*, which is quite visible to any person, when the air is moist, or of low temperature, and which ought constantly to be excreted from the lungs. This necessary process is very often retarded by the air being already charged with moisture, and its diminution of capacity to admit the vapor from the lungs; but it more frequently depends on the neglect of ventilation, and the breathing of air containing impurities, or deficient in oxygen. As the carbon can not be removed without the agency of oxygen, neither can the *hydrogen* of the blood, except it be liberated by the same agent. This hydrogen, *the water-former* (as its name implies), forms with oxygen, the watery exhalation of the breath, and like carbon can not be retained in the system with impunity.

When a sudden recession of the sensible perspiration takes place, and the minute blood-vessels of the mucous membrane lining the bowels become congested, irritation succeeds, a morbidly increased action of that canal is excited, and often results in diarrhœa, cholera, or even dysentery, all of which might have been prevented, though indirectly, by proper ventilation.

Dysentery is also often produced by the morbific agency of poisonous exhalations. "In epidemic dysentery, a peculiar disposition of the air is the reputed cause; but this can be aided by unwholesome aliment, drinks, and habitations, as with troops in camps, &c." Dewee's Practice, vol. ii., p. 569. "Miasmata have frequently an unequivocal agency, in the production of this disease. Dysentery seems indeed, very often, the production of the united influence of *koino miasmata*, and atmospheric vicissitudes." Dr. Eberle, Practice of Medicine, vol. i., p. 206. In allusion to the peculiarly fatal scorbutic dysentery, that prevailed in the Milbank Penitentiary, in England, the writer, last quoted, justly remarks: "This disease was ascribed, by the committee appointed to investigate its cause, to the constant and exclusive use of vegetable and farinaceous diet, acting in conjunction with atmospheric inclemency. I think there are good grounds for believing, that, in addition to these causes, an atmosphere inquinated with the effluvia generated, in crowded apartments, had no inconsiderable share in the production of this peculiar

11*

affection." In like manner the highest authorities, both American and European, ascribe the dysenteries of camps, ships, jails, schools, &c., more to the pollutions of the atmosphere, than to any other cause.

Dysentery sometimes prevails epidemically over large areas of country. During the summer and fall of 1848, it prevailed in a considerable degree over the northern and eastern states, and in some places was very fatal. It has repeatedly occurred endemially in some of our prisons, at times where there was no external cause for it, but at the periods of its general prevalence over the surrounding countries, the interior of a prison is very liable to become the scene of its increased malignity and fatality. Thus during its general prevalence just adverted to, at the stateprison at Sing-Sing on the Hudson river, it committed very extensive ravages. About one third of the male prisoners were attacked with it, and nearly or quite twenty fell victims to it in a short time. So in the stateprison at Auburn, it prevailed in conjunction with other symptoms of disease in the winter of 1845 and '46 to a very serious extent. The sick-list of the hospital in one year contained two hundred and ninety-two names, out of not more than six hundred prisoners, of whom twenty died; besides those who were prescribed for in their cells. In Sing-Sing, again it has happened that the medical officer has been called to render his aid to from one hundred, to one hundred and fifty cases, of this and other similar disorders, within the space of two or three days.

Although it is well-known that the character of the food used in these institutions is not such as is best calculated to promote the health of the prisoner, yet if the food, such as it is, is always administered in a sound and wholesome condition, there is no other mode of accounting for the diseases than to refer to the air of the houses, and no one, intelligent on the subject of atmospheric influences can enter those living tombs, without being immediately impressed with the idea, that few people could possibly remain long in good health in such places. The *total absence* of specific ventilation, and the consequent accumulation of the morbific effluvia from the persons contained in the narrow cells, must necessarily *often directly produce*, and *always predispose to*, diseases of various kinds, but especially such as have been mentioned.

One can not avoid the conclusion that, with the proof of the effects of confined and frequently-respired air now before the world, a heavy responsibility for the health and lives of the inmates of prisons, as well as of other places of congregation, lies upon those who are intrusted with their management, as long as they refuse or neglect to adopt the best possible means to render the *inside*, as healthful as the *outside* of their institution.

The two departments (male and female) of the state-prison at Sing-Sing, present additional evidence, if any were needed, to prove that the internal atmosphere has more to do with the production of both the chronic and acute diseases prevailing there, that any other cause, not even excepting the food. These departments occupy separate buildings. The male building is situated at the foot and on the west side of a high hill, the water of the river rising at times nearly to the level of the plane on which the foundation rests. The sun can not reach the spot till near noon for a large part of the year, and these causes, combined with the entire neglect of ventilation, maintain a constant state of moisture, very unfavorable to health.

On the other hand, the female building is placed near the brow of the hill, where the sun and air have free play, and the evils of a too moist atmosphere are not apparent. The internal ventilation is no better, though the house is, in proportion to the number of inmates, large, and less crowded. The food furnished to the two departments is the same; and though a large number of the males have the advantage over the females of working out of doors, the females being almost wholly confined within doors, yet the amount of sickness, is vastly disproportioned to their numbers; the females in general maintaining almost uninterrupted health, the labors of the physician being confined almost wholly to the male department.

There is no other satisfactory mode of accounting for the difference, than a reference to the situations and atmospheres of the two houses.

In the animal economy there is in operation a law called by physiologists "*sympathetic association.*" By this term is meant, that when any tissue or organ of the body is affected (say, for example, by irritation), all other organs connected with it are likely to be similarly affected. Thus, when the stomach is deranged, or irritated, by indigestible food, or in any other way, the brain, liver, kidneys, lungs, &c., *sympathize*, that is, become irritated also. It then follows, that if the inhalation of foul air, or its external and mechanical application, irritates and injures any part of the body, the amount of disease thus originated may become almost incalculable.

That carbonic acid, and other atmospheric adulterations, excite inflammation in the mucous membranes of the body (which line the air-passages of the lungs and those communicating in some way with the air), is a fact universally admitted. This brings us at once to the fact, that when the air-passages of the nose, throat, or lungs, are inflamed by the inhalation of carbonic acid, the other mucous membranes, and particularly that forming the external covering of the eye, must sympathize. Who has been any length of time, in a densely-crowded meeting, where ventilation was neglected, without experiencing, in some way or other, the effects here stated, and perhaps by suffering from purulent inflammation of the eye. And when air, not only highly carbonized, but also impregnated with particles of matter, some of them of a highly-irritating nature, is applied to the eye, the evil results will be doubly magnified. Entirely excluding the more unavoidable foreign bodies that mechanically injure the eye, as diet, metallic particles, animal and vegetable exhalations, &c., it is painful to contemplate how many eyes have been rendered temporarily useless, while others have become dull, lack-lustre, and expressionless, from the indulgence of those two disgusting and pernicious habits, *smoking* and *drinking*, in the act of which, generally speaking, the carbonic acid of a polluted apartment is associated with the noxious smoke of tobacco and the irritating vapor of alcohol, all of which not only tend to poison the springs of life, but concentrate their united and destructive influence, on the tenderest and most exquisitely delicate organ in the human frame. Nature, however, true to her fixed and invariable principles, resents this injury, and as the appearance of the eye is a tolerably correct exponent of the moral habits and general condition of both body and mind, it very often betrays, in a manner mortifying to its possessor, a broken constitution, and exhibits to the world, in characters that can seldom be erased from the aspect, the very habits by which moral and physical decline has been induced and perpetuated.

Many medical men, and other philanthropists, who have descended into these dens of ignorance, destitution, and distress, too common in all cities, have observed the baneful effects of impure air upon the eye, both directly and through the sympathy of the lungs, and coincide in the opinion that pure air is absolutely required by that organ for the due performance of its function.

The evidence of Mr. Toynbee before the British commission,* may be here profitably cited, as in it, the above statements are not only corroborated by a man of the most extensive experience, in the causes of the diseases of large cities, but also because it sheds considerable light on diseases arising from atmospheric impurities, which are commonly regarded as having no connexion whatever with the state of the air :—

" But do you find the operation of this one cause — the atmospheric impurity arising from overcrowding and defective ventilation — attended only by one form of disease ?"† — " The forms of scrofula, I find, are various; we have scrofulous affections of the eyes, called sore or inflamed eyes, which are very frequent ; scrofulous affections of the joints, called by the people themselves abscesses, — the abscess being in the neighborhood of the joint, and they have no idea that it communicates with the joint; this disease frequently attacks the hip-joint. The defective ventilation may be considered one great cause of all the diseases of the joints, which we so frequently meet with, as well as of the diseases of the eye and the skin; the diseases of the skin, herpetic diseases, are called shingles, lepra, porrigo, or ringworm.‡ The professional attendants of almost every eleemosynary institution, could testify to the causes as well as the prevalence of ophthalmia among the children of the poor — indeed, purulent ophthalmia (its worst form), is generally regarded as a purely scrofulous disease. The disease

---

* First Report, vol. i., p. 74.   † Scrofula.

‡ Herpetic eruptions are so called because they inclined to *creep*, as it were, or spread about the skin. This genus of disease is distinguished by an assemblage of numerous little creeping ulcers, in clusters, and itching very much, and difficult to heal, but terminating in branny scales.

of *hydrocephalus*, or water in the brain,* so fatal to children, I find associated with symptoms of scrofula, and arises in abundance in these close rooms. I believe water in the brain, in the class of patients whom I visit, to be almost wholly a scrofulous affection."†

" The general depressing influences affect most injuriously the most sensitive or weakest organs. Besides the eye, the ear is, I believe, injuriously affected by them. Among other forms of disease, which I think ascribable to the influence of vitiated air, is a large amount of what has not hitherto been ascribed to it — namely, *deafness*. In justification of this opinion, I may state, that I have already made between five and six hundred dissections of ears, with the view of determining the seat of this particular disease. One hundred and twenty of these cases I have submitted to the consideration of the profession in the 26th volume of the ' Medico Chirurgical Transactions.' The general effect observable, is the thickening of the (mucous) membrane of the middle ear. This membrane is semi-transparent, and being extremely sensitive and delicate, is, I believe, injuriously affected by the vitiated air, and debilitated by it; inflammation and other diseases are induced by the access and pressure of cold air, on leaving heated rooms, to go out into the colder atmosphere. The delicate membrane of the ear, it is to be recollected, is longer exposed to the depressing influence of the vitiated air, than any other part of the body. On leaving a room, the surface of the body is relieved

---

* More properly *water in the head*, as the effusion of water takes place, not only in the brain itself, but also very frequently in the double membrane that envelops that important organ.

† It must be kept in mind that Toynbee fully subscribes to the opinion advanced by M. Baudelocque, and which has been determined by general experience to be correct, viz , that scrofula, with its host of attendant diseases, may be produced *de novo*, by the inhalation of vitiated air alone, without hereditary taint or any other cause being necessarily present.

from the continued access of the vitiated air, while the quantity of vitiated air contained in the middle ear, remains for a considerable time, and is only slowly removed. The suspicion which I had formed from the dissections, that the cause of deafness is (occasionally), dependent upon the contact of foul air, appears to me to be corroborated by the fact that at least double the number of children of the laboring classes, are affected by earache and deafness than children of the rich and better-conditioned classes, less exposed to the like influences."

Extensive though the noxious influence of impure air may be, on the *healthy* tissues of the body, both externally and internally, it is still more so upon those diseased, or disorganized, by the effects of surgical operations. Setting aside the vitiation of the blood, and the consequent prostration of both body and mind, or the aggravation of their diseases, maladies have been produced by the direct application of vitiated air to external sores, that were sufficient to desolate whole hospitals. By the immediate action of the air of a small ill-ventilated ward, a simple abscess has been known to assume the condition of a frightful cancerous ulcer, and a mere scratch has been followed by a fatal attack of erysipelas. All the best-informed writers on *hospital gangrene*, attribute that usually fatal disease, to a corrupted atmosphere, which not only exercises a hurtful influence upon the whole animal economy when the body is afflicted with ulcers and wounds, but also by coming into direct contact with those ulcers and wounds, induces upon them a humid species of mortification, which has, generally, even under the best treatment, a fatal termination.

Wounded soldiers, and those lately operated upon, when crowded together in unhealthy encampments, especially suffer from this disease, and too often, in these cases, a familiar maxim, "The air kills more than the sword," is verified, and reduced to a terrible reality.* Hospitals were formerly so ill-ventilated, that very frequently patients were carried into them, as it were, to be poisoned by the noxious effluvia, or the carbon of their own bodies. Patients did not suffer alone. The medical attendants were carried off in great numbers. Surgeons were not more fortunate than physicians. If they did not lose their lives so frequently, they oftener lost what, perhaps, they esteemed equally precious—their reputation. Allusion is here made to the fact that very often the most skilful, dexterous, and experienced surgeon may perform on his patients, in an ill-ventilated hospital, a series of operations, all of which may be fatal to the lives of his patients, and of course fatal to his own reputation; and which might have been attended with results directly the contrary, had the wards been thoroughly ventilated.

In a case of this kind, it is an unfortunate circumstance that there are often to be found some unprincipled persons, aspiring to be members of the medical profession, but who scarcely deserve that name, who, through jealousy, very often foster the *fama clamosa* of the ignorant, who never look below the surface of things, and thus the professional reputation of many a talented individual has been unjustly tarnished or lost. Perhaps the first duty of the operating surgeon is to ascertain what provision is made to sufficiently ventilate the apartment of his patient, and postpone the use of the knife until the benefits of fresh air be guarantied without limitation; and this is his *right* as well as his *duty*.

* This is equally true with the Roman proverb : " Plures crapula quam gladius."—Gluttony kills more than the sword.

CHAPTER XI.

Influence of Impure Air on Infantile Life.—Helplessness of Infancy **not**
always Compensated for.—Negligence of Air highly Criminal.—Opinion
of Dr Clark.—Convulsions.—Dr. Duncan.—Mortality at St. Kilda.—Dr.
Ticknor.—Excessive Mortality in Dublin Hospital.—The Cause Discovered and Removed.—Infantile Mortality in Great Britain and United
States.

HITHERTO we have considered the effects of impure
air, chiefly without particular reference to age. The
general mortality at all periods of life has been already
traced, on the best authorities, to this, one of its most
potent, and most to be dreaded causes; but when we examine the operation of that cause, in the statistical records
of infantile mortality, we shall be even further aroused to
the dangerous effects of aerial poisons.

The information contained in these records will
be anticipated, when it is considered, that children,
immediately after birth, are more under the control of
the effects of air, whether pure or contaminated; that
tender, easily injured, and amenable to the injurious
influences of impure air, as the lungs, and whole constitution of adults, may be, infinitely more virulent, and
destructive, are those influences, upon beings just usher-
ed upon the stage of life, in a condition entirely more
helpless than any other species of animal. It might be
inferred from the latter circumstance that the helplessness of infancy would be compensated for by that additional care, which reasonable and intelligent creatures
are so well fitted to bestow; but alas! for the perversity

of human nature, the helplessness of childhood very often suggests to an unnatural mother, or unfeeling nurse, that the life of a *mere infant*, is only of comparative, or trifling importance; and that it is not worth while to study how much air is requisite to support its life, or how little would suspend its, as yet, feeble, and easily extinguished powers of existence.

These observations, no doubt, principally apply to the lower orders of society, especially those who are hired as out-nurses, by foundling institutions; but they also unfortunately extend to hospitals, where the children *are not* nursed out, and in many instances even to the higher and more intelligent orders of society, in which infants, through an officious, but misdirected carefulness, are deprived of the benefits of pure air, by those who are only guilty of ignorance of its value—an ignorance which, in this country where so great facilities for acquiring information exist, can not but be pronounced highly criminal.

The opinions of those who have carefully and impartially investigated this subject, and have arrived at conclusions, which our own personal experience and observation fully corroborate, will again be adduced.

" Almost all the children reared in the workhouses of this country, and in similar establishments abroad, become scrofulous, more I believe from the impure atmosphere which they breathe, and the want of sufficient exercise, than from defective nourishment."

" Take a child of three or four years of age, in perfect health, having been born without any predisposition to disease (if any such there are), well nursed, and hitherto properly nourished: let it be fed upon improper food, let it be confined to close ill-ventilated apartments, where neither the heat nor the light of the sun, has free admission, and we shall soon see the healthy blooming

child, changed into a pale, sickly, leuco-phlegmatic object."—*Dr. Clark.*

"Infancy, in particular, will fall an easy victim [to
the morbific agencies of the atmosphere]. The records
of foundling hospitals, work-houses, and other public institutions, abundantly show the injurious influence of impure air, during the periods of infancy and childhood.
One way in which it increases the mortality of infants,
is by inducing *convulsions*, in consequence of the pecu-
culiar irritability of the nervous system, at that age. In
a paper read before the medical section of the British
Association, in 1834, it was stated on the authority of the
registrar of the Lying-in Hospital, of Dublin, that in
1781, owing to the impurity of the air in the wards, 'every sixth child died within nine days after birth, of con-
vulsive disease, and that after means of thorough ventilation had been adopted, the mortality of infants in the
five succeeding years, was reduced to nearly one in
twenty.'"—*Dr. Duncan.*

When Mr. M'Clean, an intelligent Scotch writer, visited
St. Kilda, a small island on the northwest of Scotland,
he found that the population was undergoing a rapid diminution, chiefly an account of an extraordinary amount
of infantile mortality. It appeared that "eight out of
every ten died between the eighth and twelfth days of
their existence."

On looking around him for the cause of this almost
unparalleled circumstance, Mr. M'Clean found that "the
air of the island was good, and the water excellent," and
that "there was no visible defect on the part of Natuie,"
but that "the great, if not the only cause, was the filth
amid which they lived, and the *noxious effluvia* which
pervaded their houses, which it would appear, were
mere huts, small, low-roofed, and without windows."
"The clergyman," observed Mr. M'Clean, "lives exact-

ly as those around him do, in every respect, except as regards the condition of his house, and has a family of four children, the whole of whom, are well and healthy. According to the average mortality around him, three out of the four would have been dead, within the first fortnight, had he neglected cleanliness and ventilation."*

The late Dr. Ticknor, in an address to the Salisbury Lyceum, Connecticut, makes allusion to a certain pernicious nursery abuse, in the following forcible, but perfectly justifiable language: " Whether owing to our ultra-civilization, physiological refinements, or mistaken taste, or to some other cause, it matters not, if, as I believe, the condition of infancy is altogether too artificial, in regard to the contact of air. Can any mortal assign a reason for half-smothering a child in shawls and blankets, to exclude the free, pure, unadulterated, air of heaven."†

This point has been written and lectured upon centuries before the days of Ticknor, yet so deeply rooted is the prejudice, at the present day, that but a faint hope can be entertained of its removal. On the imaginations of mothers, educated as well as ignorant, the feeling still seems to be stereotyped, that the "free, pure, unadulterated air of heaven" falls upon the brow of infancy, as the poppies of eternal sleep, and enters the lungs, and circulation, as a virulent and deadly poison, and still the "shawls and blankets" sleeping and awake, are pretty generally employed to deprive the objects of the most rapturous parental solicitude, of what was originally breathed into the nostrils of the great archetype of the human race, as *"the breath of life."*

---

* " *Cleanliness*" is said to be "next to godliness," and if. after admitting this, we reflect that cleanliness can not exist without ventilation, we must then look upon the latter as not only a *moral* but a *religious* duty.

† New York Journal of Medicine, vol. ix., p. 208.

Before concluding these observations on this important topic, the probable numerical mortality among infants in this country, will be given. For this purpose, the statements of Dr. Alcott, of Boston, may be adopted, and relied upon as pretty accurate. The deaths occurring in the Dublin Lying-in Hospital, just cited, are the data upon which this writer bases his calculations. He says: " In a hospital in Dublin, between the years 1781 and 1785, no less than 2,944 children out of 7,650 died within a fortnight after their birth. This was more than one in three. Dr. Clark, the physician, suspecting the cause to be a want of air, contrived to introduce a full supply of this important element, by means of pipes, six inches in diameter, into all the apartments. The consequence was, that during the three succeeding years only 165 out of 4,243 children died within the first two weeks, or less than one in twenty-five. What a surprising difference! Is there a doubt that of the first number of deaths we have mentioned, about 2,650 died for want of pure air ?

" According to the best information we are able to obtain on the subject, about forty in every one hundred of the deaths annually occurring in Great Britain and the United States, are of children under five years of age. To avoid every possibility of exaggeration, we will, however, place the number in the United States at thirty in one hundred. But even at this rate, we lose no less than 150,000 children under five years of age every year. Now if the infantile mortality, was reduced in the Dublin hospital, from one in three to one in twenty-five, merely by supplying them with an abundance of pure air ; that is, if the attention paid to this single department of health was the means of saving young infants, there, at the rate of 130,000 in 150,000, is it too much to believe, that at least 50,000 of those who die annually in the United States, under the age of five years, might be saved in the same way. We do not, of course, mean to affirm that the exact number of 50,000 children, and no more, actually die, annually, in the United States, for want of pure air. It may be more, it may be less. Some thousands, — nay some tens of thousands, — however, it must be. But this is not all. Thousands, and tens of thousands of others, whose lives extend beyond this period, are yet sufferers from the same cause; and though their natural force of constitution may enable them to live on a little longer than those whose constitutions are more feeble, yet are they not more to be pitied ?"*

* Health Tracts.—" Breathing Pure Air."

CHAPTER XII.

Present Condition and Prospects of Society in Relation to Health and Civilization.

Iτ is difficult to determine or define the present condition of society, as compared with that existing in the early ages· of the world — whether advancing or retrograding in civilization, properly so called — whether improving or degenerating, in physical or mental energy. This question is not to be decided by theory or speculation, but by facts only. Men's ideas of civilization, and their sanatory condition, like their ideas of religion, fashion, beauty, &c., are as various as their physiognomical appearances. Some are prone to embrace the darkest side of the question, without appealing to any data upon which they can build their opinions, while others run into the opposite extreme, and embrace the most hopeful aspect of affairs, and take their safety upon trust, without inquiring if the danger be removed. Some of the latter will, for example, assert that physical and mental energy are on the increase, and as a proof, point to what they call " *the increased value of human life.*" However specious this reasoning may appear, it is fallacious. The facts that have been brought forward, stubbornly oppose such a doctrine. Even if it were satisfactorily proved, which it is not, that the average duration of life is on the increase, we are not therefore warranted in supposing that the human race has not degenerated. It is quite possible that man may be less vigorous in every respect now, than in ancient times, and yet be longer-lived; and it is absurd to assume the mystical calculations of a Roman judge, grounded, as they were, on the longevity of the Romans, when their degeneration was nearly complete, as a standard by which to judge the sanatory condition and longevity of *all* the ancients. The Romans were then in the same transition state of moral, social, economical, and physical decline, that impends many nations now existing, which have by adopting an imperfect social structure, subjected themselves to the same causes; with perhaps this difference, that the Romans were too far advanced before they saw their error, to recover themselves by a *sanatory regeneration*. Many causes operated to curtail the lives of the ancients, which do not now exist — and these causes themselves sprung from a superior physical and mental development.

Men in former times, recklessly embarked in any exploit, no matter how dangerous, spurred on by the strong but misdirected impulse of mental and physical power. Almost every man, at sometime or other of his life, risked it in the battlefield, and as war was a universal trade, many lost their lives in their prime. Besides, the people were almost universally ignorant of the means of preserving health, and restoring it when lost, and quackery, ignorance, and superstition, either directly or indirectly, swept off the diseased in numbers unparalleled in the annals of modern mortality. Now, millions live without ever risking their lives beyond the little circle of accidents that of necessity surrounds them, and as a general rule, never expose themselves to danger because they instinctively know they have not the fortitude to brave it, or the power to ward it off, or resist it. In this way, their carefulness of life and health has increased, but this carefulness has by no means kept pace with the danger. On the subject of Hygiene, they have attained to an *intelligence*, but it is not yet matured into an *edu-*

cated intelligence. At mid-life, they find themselves afflicted with chronic diseases, and premature decrepitude;
they have, however, learned to nurse themselves into a
sere old age, which would have been abridged by many
years, had they been exposed to the dangers and fatigues
of their ancestors. They have still to learn how to nurse
themselves into health, and *prevent* this premature decrepitude.

A priori, we should expect, that what with refinements
in every department of knowledge, and the general absence of the influences lately specified, our health would
be better and our term of existence much longer; but
this has not been proved. On the contrary, it is found,
that the number of centenaries is in reputedly civilized
countries yearly growing smaller, and health on the
decline. Nations still almost primitive in their way
of living, we would also expect to be delicate, diseased,
and short-lived. A visit to the North American Indians,
to many of the South-sea islanders, or even to the
Hottentots and Patagonians, would soon undeceive us,
and convince us of the contrary. To say that these
men are stupid, or void of mental culture, does not in
any way invalidate the original proposition, as *strength*
or rather *material* of mind is only contended for, and as
to their health of both body and mind, this is a fact which
is not attempted to be denied.

It is quite clear that society is constructed on erroneous principles, as erroneous indeed as the architectural
arrangement and structure of the houses of its members.
Both are built up without reference to health. It is also
clear that its sacred destiny must yet be fulfilled, although
it is now on the wane, and tending toward what would
seem its final extinction. It must therefore be in its
destiny to be regenerated, and this is now evidently prac-
ticable. Many causes of degeneracy have been pointed

out by late writers, who are competent judges, as may be seen in the extracts in the past pages. Plans have been pointed out for the removal of many of these causes, and some have been removed. This is cheering, but still men, women, and children, and even the lower animals, are yearly dying by millions, for want of fresh air, and many other causes; but the increase of those causes, has hitherto more than counter-balanced the success of any attempts that have been made to remove them. Though the thread of human life is nearly as extended as former-ly, it has become alarmingly more tiny and delicate, and more easily snapped; and though the human species have rapidly increased in numbers, their physical and mental energy, have almost as rapidly diminished. Some say we are *ultra-civilized,* but that contradiction in terms, should only be meant as a degeneration of society, and in that sense only is it admissible. True civilization can only be reached, when the sanatory condition of society is on the progressive.

A *sanatory regeneration* of society should now be the object of all its members, and one aim of their exertions. Many are no doubt ignorant, and the great bulk of so-ciety apathetic; but it is, as has been said, cheering, that a revolution of sentiment has commenced. Howards are springing up in many places, who are not afraid to risk their health, and even their lives, to redeem the health and vigor of their fallen race, and sublimate it to its des-tined perfection. All their admonitions and exertions will be useless, and their legal enactments inoperative, or ineffective, unless the people co-operate. This they will not do except they understand the benefits of those measures, and these they will not understand, until they be educated;—educated physically, educated morally, educated intellectually, educated religiously, or, in short, *educated physiologically.* How can they be expected to appreciate pure air, for example, until they have learned and understood its value. The first step to be secured, the vantage ground to be gained, is to recover by a perfect system of education, and wise sanatory laws, that energy of body and mind which were possessed and often perverted by the ancients; the energy that gave birth to the invincible fortitude, warlike spirit, and chivalry of the olden time; to bring back the energy whether uselessly wasted on those monuments of folly we see scattered up and down, or profitably employed in the pursuits of sciences, to generalize that energy which lately deluged in blood, the streets of the most polished city in the world, a city which has assumed the attitude of the centre point and climax of civilization; to first attain to this energy *without* the wickedness and vanity to which, when perverted, it gives rise. Then we would have gained the material out of which to elaborate a structure of society, of body and of mind, as perfect as is possible in our temporal state. Then we would be in the fair way of achieving the *sanatory regeneration* of the human race. Then our bodies, our minds, our houses, our cities, our communities, our whole social fabric, would be, in the course of being, rebuilt on a sure foundation.

CHAPTER XIII.

Modern Degeneracy of the Human Race.—Superior Vigor of the Ancient Egyptians, Athenians, and Romans.—Inaptitude for Study an Effect of Vitiated Air.—Newton.—Homer.—Sleeping in Church—Anecdote.—Perversion of Judgment.—Extract from Dr. Ticknor.—Vitiated Air produces Quarrelsomeness—encourages Intemperance, and other Vices —also Pusillanimity and Cowardice, and vice versa.—Examples.—True Courage, where to be found.—Defective Ventilation increases Public Expenditure.—Produces Deformity, Imbecility, and Idiotcy.—Cretinism.—A Mournful Picture.—Found in Cellars of Cities.—Idiots in France, Turkey, and other Countries.—Changes in the Earth and in Man, Compared.

For many centuries past, we have had numerous writers and preachers on the moral degeneracy of mankind, and many still are asserting, on spiritual grounds, the increasing laxity and gradual decline of morals, and the growing disregard of strict principles of religion and rectitude. But it must strike us forcibly, that though physical degeneracy has also been making equally rapid strides, and progressing hand in hand with moral decay, it was not until very lately, that those who are the properly-constituted guardians of health, have raised their voices, or taken up their pens, to arrest its progress. That this degeneracy actually exists, and is still progressive, is not a subject of controversy, but capable of easy demonstration. A glance back at the history of the world, and the contrast that presents itself between the mental, moral, and physical condition of society in ages long past, and

13

its condition as regards these relations, now, is met by a sudden and humiliating conviction of the awful dilapidation that has taken place in the social fabric. It is impossible for the present age to flatter itself into the contrary opinion. As the accumulation of literature, which is stored up in the huge intellectual magazine into which the world has grown, and the multiplied facilities of modern education, which a long experience has secured, are no proofs that we are relatively increasing in strength of mind; so our concentrated facilities and stupendous triumphs of bodily labor, are no proofs that we are relatively increasing in physical energy. On the contrary, when we look back with an impartial eye on the severe and unbending morality, the refinement in taste and sentiment, the mental and physical vigor, so common among the ancient Egyptians, Athenians, and Romans, as evinced, at the present day, in monuments which have defied the wreck of time and the vandalism of ages, and then make allowance for our advantages, we are penetrated with an irresistible sense of relative inferiority, and can no longer boast of our march of intellect, and our splendid achievements. Under these circumstances, it is clearly the duty of every member of society to exert any influence he may happen to possess, to avert this impending calamity, and if he have a mite of information on its removable causes, to give it free publicity.

Taking it for granted that the startling facts and arguments, adduced and authenticated in the preceding pages, have already established the conviction that adulterated air is one of the most fertile sources of physical degeneracy, we shall now proceed to show that the same cause, of itself, or as an auxiliary, is capable of producing a still more grievous degeneracy of the mind, and total depravation of man as a social, moral, and intellectual being.

With the spirituality of the subject, we of course have

nothing to do, as the duty of its exposition legitimately belongs to the province of others, and we will only consider man in his moral and mental capacity, and influenced by physical causes.

The following are some of the more ordinary effects of vitiated air upon the mind and morals:—

1st. *Vitiated air produces inaptitude for study, and therefore ignorance.* This may be observed in any ill-ventilated school or seminary, and instances are too numerous for citation. It is well-known that sometime previous to dismission, the pupils are sluggish and languid in both body and mind, and the accumulation of carbon and its inhalation, greatly incapacitate for any serious study. Even the eye becomes irritated by its contact with the impurities of the air, and by its sympathy with the brain, and while it loathes the fatiguing sameness of the print and paper, longs to refresh itself on the green variegated carpet of nature. The wholesome regulation of allowing the children to retire after each lesson, in classes, for a short time to the play-ground, is to be highly commended, as it is based on the correct and rational principle, that when the cerebral functions become weakened by inefficient respiration, the mind can only be invigorated by a due supply of pure air and exercise, after which it returns to its work with renewed ardor, and redeems by redoubled energy and success, that time which the managers and teachers of some schools would ignorantly suppose to be squandered away. On the other hand, when children are confined long hours in an ill-ventilated school, the incipient symptoms of poisoning by carbonic acid, viz.: headache, languor, debility, and irritability, will ensue, and these, kept up for a considerable time, rarely fail to produce diseases, which permanently impair the body and mind, and which can not afterward be eradicated from the constitution of either.

It has also been observed that children contract a dull idle disposition, and become quite averse to habits of order, cleanliness, and industry.

Those who studied or composed in the open air, were the greatest and most successful thinkers of ancient and modern times. Sir Isaac Newton made his greatest discovery while in a garden, where he was wont to pursue his studies. The peripatetics, perhaps the most enlightened philosophers of their age, used to *walk up and down* in the porches of the Lyceum, at Athens, and it is said—

> " Seven cities contend for Homer, dead,
> Through which the living Homer begged his bread;"

from which it may be inferred, that one of the most exalted productions of human intellect, was composed when its illustrious author was journeying from place to place in the open air.—Similar examples are numberless.

On the other hand, when children are, as it were, incarcerated in a school-room for many hours together, and exposed to the effects of carbon, it makes them as incapable of mental as of physical exertion; and languor and lassitude being incompatible with the healthy operation of the mind, ignorance and its concomitant evils, are the results. These effects are not more strikingly observable in school-rooms, than in lecture-rooms of colleges, private studies, court-rooms, churches, public assemblies, theatres, &c., in which there is inadequate ventilation. Alas! how many young men, who might, under favorable circumstances, have become ornaments and benefactors to their adopted professions and to society at large, have been stupified into ignorance; or who, by hard study under the slow and insidious influence of carbonic acid, have heaped up loads of erudition alike useless to themselves and to others, and speedily paid the debt of Nature, while they paid the penalty of infringing the unchangeable laws of their own organs, in neglecting to keep úp health of body while they were storing the mind.

The pulpit orator too, finds that his midnight lucubrations, manufactured while he is cooped up within the precincts of a study which is small, ill-ventilated, and hampered with books and manuscripts, will often fail to charm his audience, especially when they are nodding under the influence of the densely-carbonized atmosphere of an ill-ventilated church.

An anecdote very illustrative of this, is related of an old Scottish pulpit orator, of a standing above mediocrity for eminence and ability, who was so mortified and annoyed at the unaccountable apathy, inattention, and drowsiness of his hearers, that he deemed it expedient to preach a series of sermons on " *The sin and shame o' sleepin' in kirkes.*" This resolution was carried out with an extraordinary fervor and force of argument, but without any appreciable effect. His lions and angels neither roused the fears, nor excited the admiration of his seemingly lukewarm flock, and the flowers of his eloquence only "lost their sweetness on the [poisoned] air." There one sat yawning with his eyes half-closed, his face flushed, head aching, and languor and mental inactivity evident on his countenance, which also indicated a partial unconsciousness of his own existence. Here another, in the corner, with his forehead lazily resting on the back of the pew before him, enjoying a rather comfortable nap, interrupted though it was by his having occasionally to raise his head, to show the pastor and those around him, that he was not absolutely sleeping.

At last, a thought fortunately crossed the preacher's mind : that a mouthful or two of fresh air, might possibly have some beneficial effect, in stimulating the mental appetite, and keeping up attention. The sexton was accordingly ordered to throw the windows partially open

13*

during the hours of service. The experiment was attended with complete success, and tended greatly to improve the understanding between the pastor and his flock.

2d. *That the judgment is perverted to a certain extent*, and the mind thwarted from its original object, by the frequently-respired air of a crowded assembly, there is good show of reason. Dr. Ticknor, in his address to the Salisbury Lyceum,* says: " The impurity of air once, or more than once, inspired, is not acknowledged by the senses, but is *felt* by the lungs and brain. If such impurities possessed visible qualities, we should often, I fancy, be frightened from crowded rooms and close sleeping apartments. From the first to the last inspiration, a pure atmosphere is more essential to the health of body and mind than you may suppose. A slight diminution of oxygen in the air, such as would result from half a dozen of persons in the room, is distressingly obvious to an asthmatic, or others who have suffered a destruction of some portion of the lungs. Perhaps there is nothing more true, and perhaps nothing less observed, in relation to this subject than this, namely, that the high excitement, occasionally manifesting itself in fierce language, ending in personal injury and homicide; involving consequences most disastrous to individuals, families, and communities, is frequently more the result of physical than moral causes. This may be *too strong* an assertion; take another—the moral causes would not often show such results, without the co-operation of the physical. I mean a raised temperature of a very frequently-respired atmosphere. What think you would have been the effect of a fresh northeast wind upon our patriotism, unbroken by boards and shingles at our late election ? Why our love of country would not have come so near personal hatred and personal abuse. I would not offend, but speak I

* New York Journal of Medicine, Vol. XX., No. xxvi., p. 209.

must, and speak I will, on this subject. The enthusiasm, the burning, blustering patriotism, by which our great gatherings are characterized, are to a great extent the effects of an atmosphere loaded with carbonic acid and other impurities, rather than a just appreciation of our country's wants and her claims upon us. This doctrine is true as far as its application to the lower animals can be made. Those of a combative character, when crowded together, become quarrelsome and destroy each other. I would recommend, therefore, when health of body and mind is the thing desired, that a moderate temperature and absolutely pure state of the air be maintained."

These observations may seem for the moment, overworked, but on mature reflection they will be found to be judicious, and based upon facts almost daily escaping observation.

3d. *Vitiated air encourages intemperance in the use of intoxicating drinks.* Among the various causes which excite a morbid appetite for these liquors, is found an atmosphere that depresses the spirits, and thus creates a demand for some stimulant to restore the brain to its former action. Pure air would now be the natural and proper stimulant, without producing a short-lived and boisterous hilarity, but in the midst of a smoky city, with a limited time for recreation, and with a feebleness of body as well as mind, occasioned by hard work or unremitted attention to business, in an ill-ventilated workshop, or counting-house, the artisan or clerk has neither inclination nor ability to avail himself of the more rational and invigorating relaxations, and resorts to the punch and oyster saloon, or liquor store, to procure the most likely means of affording to the debilitated organs a temporary relief. A habit is thus established which is at best a delusion, fatal to the health and morals; and which not only defeats its own object, but aggravates the evil it is in-

tended to remove; the ultimate effect of every fit of in-
toxication, or even exhilaration of mind brought on by
alcoholic drinks, being to precipitate and degrade the
mind and habits, to a point still lower in the scale of
demoralization and degeneracy.

Even children, whose nervous systems have been work-
ed up into a state of chronic excitability by the impure
air of a dark ill-ventilated cellar, are often dosed with
spirits, when laudanum is not at hand, to put them to
sleep and abridge the *trouble* of nurses and mothers.

This erroneous and cruel practice not only defeats its
own object, but what is worse, instils into plastic and susceptible youth, habits which, as they obscure the reason
and bias the judgment, will seldom be relinquished in
maturity or old age.

4th. *Impure air encourages vice.* Vice, and habits of in-
toxication, are usually combined in the same individual.
If, then, it has been already shown that impure air
promotes drunkenness, it is also indirectly proved that
the same cause has a considerable share in the encouragement of vice. The inhabitants of low, squalid, ill-
ventilated basements and cellars, are often not only indisposed, but by incessantly breathing an impure atmosphere are actually unable to labor for their due support; add to this the mental debility, and extinction of
moral sentiments, inseparable from a cellar life, and we
at once arrive at *one* of the efficient causes of poverty, of
low ideas of comfort, and of dishonesty, and prostitution;
and as it is notorious that, in such places, intoxicating drinks
are held in higher estimation than any of the virtues, it is
nothing strange to hear of modesty being set to sale for the
acquirement of those drinks, which in their turn reciprocally produce every conceivable species of moral laxity.

But impure air has even more direct effects in producing and fostering vice, and it is only because this

work is intended to be popular that the opinions of several eminent pathologists on this point are suppressed.

The combined testimony of those who have taken the pains to investigate the causes of vice and prostitution, leaves no doubt that a low condition of body and mind, coincident with a morbid irritability of the brain, so far from restraining (as might be surmised) the animal propensities and vicious inclinations, has no inconsiderable share in their aggravation and production ; and this position being granted, ample evidence, it is presumed, has been adduced to show that the impure air of factories, theatres, over-crowded lodging-houses, &c., is fully adequate to induce this state of constitution.

5th. *Vitiated air encourages pusillanimity and cowardice.* This position may seem to many, strange, if not untenable. Some of the German writers hold the opinion that the inhabitants of mountainous and high lying countries, are, from the greater purity of the air, vivacious, " friendly and hilarious," while those of the low lying countries are more sullen and unfriendly.*

The history of nations not only corroborates this opinion, but carries it further. The boldest and most warlike nations, are generally to be found in the most mountainous countries, and in barbarous ages when no education controlled the feelings, propensities, and passions of men, and when the problem " what constitutes true bravery" had not yet been solved, we find them the terror of their more effeminate and pusillanimous neighbors who occupied the plains below. As examples, Wallace was inspired with confidence when he was surrounded by the " sons of the mountain glen," and Tell looked with equal pride on his valiant followers and the crags and cliffs which gave them birth, and from the

* Vide Baron Feuchtersleben's " Medical Psychology," edition of the Sydenham Society, p. 171.

free and unpolluted air of whose sides, they had imbibed their physical strength and unshrinking fortitude.

It is not of course intended here to sympathize in that barbarous spirit, which prompts men to shed the blood of their neighbors, even though they may be their enemies; but these examples are designed to show that the *material* of intellectual excellence, liberty, magnanimity, and moral courage, is more likely to be found, and developed by education, in situations where the air is uncontaminated, than in the vitiated atmosphere of a marsh; in well-ventilated mansions, than in the dark garrets and those low soul-degrading and pestiferous dens of carbonic acid and other aeriform hydras from which fresh air, true bravery, and every other noble and patriotic sentiment, are simultaneously excluded.

To find true courage it is not necessary to visit the battle-field. As bright, if not brighter, examples are to be found in the humble cot. The industrious housewife exhibits more true courage in retrenching the half of her daily food, to feed her hungry children, and to buy soap to wash their clothes and her own, than an Alexander, a Cæsar, a Bonaparte, or some of our own illustrious heroes, ever displayed. This woman, indeed, exhibits true magnanimity: but supposing this amiable aspiration, viz., to bring her children up in the greatest possible comfort, order, industry, and cleanliness, on the scanty means within her reach—suppressed by any cause, say by carbonic acid, a sedative poison, sedative for industry, perseverance, and all the social and domestic virtues— then, her magnanimity is immediately transformed into carelessness, apathy, and moral cowardice. As she has now lost her self-dependence, which was formerly the mainspring of her happiness, so have her children, who have copied her feelings and habits. Her husband also, breathing the same polluted atmosphere, during his hours of sleep, with nothing but filth before his eyes while under his own roof, soon becomes enervated and feeble in body and mind, he *will not, can not work.* He has now, neither moral fortitude, nor muscular ability; he is not now ashamed to ask relief. The whole family are cast upon the charity of others; perhaps, of the very men whose ignorance or negligence produced the evil. They are now pauperized, their independence of mind is extinguished—they are slaves.—Thus it is that *defective ventilation unnecessarily increases the public expenditure.*

6th. *Vitiated air produces deformity, imbecility, and idiocy.* It has been already shown, on the authority of M. Baudelocque, and others, that scrofula is often the direct result of vitiated air. Bronchocele, or goitre, hydrocephalus, and cretenism, are endemial in those districts where the air is confined, and there is now little doubt, that scrofula and its *suite* of physical, mental, and moral ailments, originate very often in deep narrow mountain gorges, and are thence propagated by intermarriages, and hereditary taint, to more salubrious districts, or to garrets and basements, where the impure air facilitates their development; as well as produces it *de novo.* Baudelocque's explanation of the condition of the air, in certain of these situations, constitutes at least the most plausible theory of the origin of these diseases, if it is not tantamount to a proof.

" There are countries," says Baudelocque, " where, independent of the mode of living of the inhabitants, scrofula is endemic. This is owing to locality. This is the case with villages built in the narrow gorges, formed by the approach of elevated mountains, as is seen in the Alps and Pyrenees, and especially in those of the valley of the Rhone. The air respired habitually in these gorges is *stagnant, humid, warm,* and corrupt; its renewal is very difficult. Ordinarily, this renewal can only be effected by the displacement of the upper strata, which are continually affected by the winds. Occasionally, the direction of the wind corresponds with the line of the gorge; and then, there is a more rapid and effectual renewal. But there always remains a part, which, being arrested by the bottom of the gorge, is, as it were, heaped back upon itself, momentarily compressed, but not displaced, and therefore, not renewed.

"The renewal of the air, is not so light a matter as is supposed. To effect it, a simple communication is not sufficient, a mere contact of the external and internal air. It is necessary that one or more *currents* exist, to multiply that contact, and cause the pure air to pervade that which is vitiated. I believe one of the principal offices of the winds, is to maintain the uniform composition of the air, by continually agitating it, so as to mingle that which has lost a part of its oxygen with that which is surcharged."

In fact, there are insuperable difficulties in the way of supposing that the winds could possibly produce an effectual renewal of the air, in the bottoms of some of the valleys, and when it is considered that *cretinism* is most prevalent in such places, — that a scrofulous condition, perfectly analogous, has been occasionally produced in vaults and prisons, where the air was confined — that facts are wanting to prove its origin from any other cause (though other causes may aggravate it when produced), the validity of Baudelocque's conclusions may be safely admitted.

The following description of the Cretins, inhabiting some of the gorges in the Alps, and which will serve for those miserable caricatures of humanity as they are found in many other countries, is taken from the pen of Dr. J. Johnson, and constitutes a powerful illustration of the horrors of vitiated air.

It will, in fact, show, in almost as strong language as can be employed, that atmospheric impurities are capable of degrading man to the lowest deep to which he can, in his present state, be precipitated.

" Goitre, on such a scale as we see in the Vallais, is bad enough, but CRETINISM is a cure for the pride of man, and may here* be studied by the philosopher and the physician on a large scale, and in its most frightful colors. This dreadful deformity of body and mind is not confined to the Alps. It is seen among the Pyrenees — the valleys of the Tyrol — and the mountains of China and Tartary. Nearly two hundred years have elapsed since it was noticed by Plater, in the spot where I am now viewing it ; but Saussure was the first who accurately described the terrible degeneracy of the human species. From common bronchocele (goitre), and a state of body and mind bordering on health, down to a complete destitution of intelligence and sensibility — in short, to an existence purely vegetative — Cretins present an infinite variety of intermediate grades, filling up these wide extremes. In general, but not invariably, goitre is an attendant on cretinism. The stature is seldom more than from four to five feet, often much less — the head is deformed in shape, and too large in proportion to the body — the skin is yellow, cadaverous, or of a mahogany color, wrinkled, sometimes of an unearthly pallor, with unsightly eruptions — the flesh is soft and flabby — the tongue is large, and often hanging out of the mouth — the eyelids thick — the eyes red, prominent, watery, and frequently squinting — the countenance void of all expression except that of idiotism or lasciviousness — the nose flat — the mouth large, gaping, slavering, the lower jaw elongated — the belly pendulous — the limbs crooked, short, and so distorted as to prevent anything but a wad-

* Sion.

14

dling progression — the external senses often imperfect, and the Cretin deaf and dumb; — the *tout ensemble* of this hideous abortion of nature presenting the traits of premature old age! Such is the disgusting physical exterior of the apparently wretched, but perhaps comparatively happy, Cretin!"

" If we look to the moral man (if man he can be called), the picture is still more humiliating. The intellectual functions being, as it were, null, certain of the lower animal functions are in a state of increased activity. The Cretins are voracious, and are addicted to low propensities, which can not be named. To eat and to sleep form their chief pleasures. Hence we see them between meals basking in nonchalance on the sunny sides of the houses, insensible to every stimulus that agitates their more intelligent fellow-creatures — frequently insensible to every call of nature itself."*

Here we have a picture of the effects of impure air, when its impurities are concentrated and localized, and when they have been inhaled without intermission — drawn from the life. It would probably be no easy task to convince the inhabitants of more genial climes that such evils existed among themselves in a more subdued form; yet such is the fact.

The Swiss peasant, inhabiting one of these reservoirs of pestilence, can not, like one of our peasants or laborers, emancipate himself from the loathsome atmosphere of an ill-ventilated bedroom, to breathe the salubrious air of the fields and groves; he can not give his semistagnant circulation even a moment's respite, by unloading it, in any degree, of its poisonous and redundant accumulations. Thus he feels the brunt of those impurities more severely, and they are more strongly developed

---

* Change of Air and Philosophy of Travelling, by J, Johnson, M. D., p. 62.

in his bodily appearance and intellect.   But this circumstance is no encouragement for the inhabitants of more
favored localities to think themselves entirely exempted
from cretinism.   So far from this being the case, they
will find that cretinism, in its incipient state, exists to an
awful extent among the cellar and garret population of
many of the large European and American cities.   Indeed, the existence of many of its characteristic symptoms (as hydrocephaloid complaints, &c.), have been already, in the foregoing pages, traced in those places, and
from a similar cause.   If the inquiry should be instituted,
Why are idiocy and mania more prevalent in the polished and civilized than in the semi-civilized and barbarous nations? — Why, for example, are there one hundred idiots and maniacs in France for one in Turkey?
One thousand in France, England, and America for one
among the Hottentots and Patagonians, in proportion to
their numbers — it would transpire that bad air, inseparable from the habits of the people, and their erroneous
principles of civilization, are among the most active
causes of this social calamity.   As a further confirmation
of the identity of these complaints, many have been
cured of mental aberration and insanity, by simple removal to fresh air, in the same way as the Swiss peasant,
when he sees cretinism setting in among his children,
immediately elevates them, if his means will allow, to the
free atmosphere of the mountain's brow, when, if the
malady has not advanced too far, they soon begin to re-
assume the image of their Creator.

The physical and moral revolutions of the world, have,
as it were, swept over it unnoticed.   Time, so gradual in
its operations, works so slowly, that a revolution is accomplished before it is observed.   Valleys have become hills,
and hills have become valleys, before the phenomena at-
tracted attention.   Towns which at the birth of Christ

were maritime, and of great commercial importance, are now inconsiderable villages, from fifteen to twenty miles from the sea! So it is with the physical and mental constitution of man. A quiet and regular succession of changes have occurred to both his body and mind, which have escaped the notice of those who have not exercised a strict investigation. The air itself may have been possibly an imperceptible medium, or instrument of his improvement, and possibly the medium or instrument of his transformation into a being inferior to the original standard of the human race.

CHAPTER XIV.

Increased Influence of Foul Air during Sleep.—Boarding-Schools.—Soldiers in Barracks.—Seamen—Nightmare prevalent among them.—Obscurity of its depredations.—Bad Air not less active, because invisible——Universal study of Physiology urged.—Sleeping with the Head covered.—Its Deleterious Effects.—Cutaneous Exhalation of Carbonic Acid.—Appalling Disaster in 1848.

One of the most insidious means by which impure air, or inefficient respiration, assails the happiness, and undermines the health, of mankind, is through the action of the superabundant carbon upon the brain, during sleep.

The misery and disease which this single cause inflicts upon the human race, exceed credibility, unless the reciprocal sympathy existing between the lungs and the brain, or in other words, between the respiratory and cerebral functions, be duly estimated and understood.

The proximate cause of sleep is still a subject of speculation, but physiologists seem to be agreed that one of the most essential conditions to the due performance of this important function, is the maintenance of an exact *equilibrium* in the amount of oxygenated blood transmitted to the brain. Whenever this equilibrium is disturbed by imperfect aeration, sleep must be disturbed also, and every person knows that insufficient or disturbed sleep, operating for even a short time, is often followed by results the most disastrous to the general constitution. The most careless observer, the hard-working day-laborer, for example, who never in his life

14*

heard of such a thing as oxygen, though he has lived upon it all his days — who has no dread whatever of carbonic acid, though it is perhaps his greatest enemy — who seldom recollects that there is such a thing as air at all — must have remarked, that he has never slept soundly in an ill-ventilated chamber, the atmosphere of which was probably charged (as is often the case) with the excrementitious and poisonous exhalations of a dozen pairs of lungs. Granted, that his body has been fatigued, and his muscular system exhausted, by continued physical exertion, possibly under the rays of a scorching sun — that his mind is untroubled — that the " *wear and tear*" of his whole system has imperatively demanded rest and renovating slumber — in short, that all the conditions necessary to the proper exercise of this peculiar function of the brain, be present, except ventilation — he rises in the morning languid and unrefreshed, and with the expression of fatigue ineffaced from his countenance.

No doubt the carbonic acid may occasionally produce a torpor, by no means disagreeable, for the time, and sometimes intense torpidity, but this state is uniformly followed by a depression, and morbid excitability of the nervous system, totally incompatible with the restoration of its energy, and the necessary recruitment of the muscular powers. An impeded respiration during sleep, no matter how occasioned, always produces anxiety and restlessness, that are followed up during the day with languor, and lassitude of both body and mind; and those who through ignorance, imprudence, or necessity, indulge in the practice of sleeping in an atmosphere highly carbonized, or loaded with other impurity, may prepare themselves for a whole catalogue of diseases, and possibly, among their other calamities, to be nightly haunted with unwelcome and debilitating dreams, idle phantasies, and dangers which will soon be realized in the form of nightmare, melancholia, and a host of other distressing nervous maladies.

Any person who may profess himself skeptical as to the activity here ascribed to atmospheric impurities, in disturbing the function of sleep, would do well to visit, some morning, the dormitories of boarding-houses and boarding-schools, where many individuals pass the night together, in the same crowded apartments, and by carefully scanning the countenances of their occupants, and inquiring into the amount of renovation derived from the past night's sleep, he would obtain some useful information. In effect, the usual answer would be, we sank "to rest, but not to sleep," perhaps to neither. But if this test should still seem unsatisfactory, and the foregoing observations wiredrawn, or gratuitous, it would perhaps suffice to inspire conviction, if he should next put his inquiries to soldiers in crowded encampments, or seamen (say the sailors of the port of New York), men who, of all others, are most exposed, especially in winter, to carbonic acid during the night. In the larger navies, the American especially, this evil is remedied, to some extent, by partial ventilation. Even in a few merchant-vessels some steps have been taken in the right direction, and an approximate improvement effected, but the vast majority of the coasting-vessels in this country, a great number of those employed for the purposes of emigration, and almost all vessels engaged in the coal-trade in Great Britain and Ireland, afford the most appalling examples of discomfort, in regard to the forecastles and other places appropriated to the seamen's berths and hammocks.

No men require more refreshing sleep than sailors, as their work is particularly exhausting, their time for that purpose uncertain, and usually limited to a few hours; yet they are generally ready to acknowledge that their rest is greatly embarrassed and disturbed, though they do not always understand the cause; and it is a fact (noticed by Waller) that in no class of men is *nightmare* more prevalent; and that among their other diseases, arising from a similar cause, none stands more prominent than the mental perturbations that afflict them during sleep, and unfit them for their duty while awake.

If there can be any palliation or excuse for the wide-spread inattention to the dangers of carbonic acid, it is to be found in the reflection, that this great cankerworm seldom makes its depredations openly upon the surface of society, but that it preys upon its vitals unobserved, begins first at the core, and not, like most of the other foes to human health and happiness, exerting its fatal influences with equal malignity, whether its victims be sleeping or awake. The drunkard, for example, is conscious that he is entailing disease and misery upon himself and his family, while the alcohol which he has adopted as his poison, besides being a tangible object, and possessing many attractions to his depraved taste and appetite, makes him reel and stagger, and exhibits to the world, in the most unequivocal symptoms, its peculiar effects upon his constitution and circumstances. But the slow and gradual poison of carbonic acid covers its approaches, and secretly and silently saps the constitution of the teetotaler as well as the intemperate, of the industrious laborer as well as the spendthrift, of infancy and youth as well as old age, of the rich as well as the indigent, and in too many instances, of the learned, as of the ignorant.

This inattention, and its attendant mischiefs, will of course continue to a variable extent, until all classes in the community have learned to know themselves, and the moral sentiment, " *nosce teipsum* ' be fully appreciated, and made the groundwork of public and private instruction. In fact, people seem to be generally unaware, in regard to atmospheric impurities, that an invisible cause is capable of producing a visible effect, and because they do not *see* that cause, they need not dread its effects.* This error of judgment is the more glaring and inconsistent, as they are in the habit of admitting the former principle, and rejecting the latter, in almost every other department of philosophy.

But the remedy is at hand. Physiology, popularized, and with certain limitations, must be made a branch of elementary instruction in all schools and seminaries, and be looked upon as an indispensable ingredient in the education of every laborer and mechanic. Great credit is due to many enlightened and benevolent persons in this country, for the influence they have brought to bear on this important point, and for the encouragement they have latterly given to the study of physiology in the elementary schools. In the great majority of them, however, the children have no information whatever on the subject. They are not even taught the simple axiom, that air is at least as necessary to their existence as food, and that food would be of no service to them without air. Examples of this rad-

---

* " In Strath we literally breathed the liquid sunshine ; but in cities the want of ventilation at our churches and chapels is a serious grievance ; and an eminent chemist, wishing lately to prove what a poisonous atmosphere is endured by crowded congregations, in Edinburgh, carefully bottled off a specimen of the air of various churches, after the audience had dispersed. The result was, that a fly could scarcely survive upon the polluted air which had been breathed successively by a dozen of persons, at least, or if the sermon has been long, by double the number. I often wish that air might become dyed of a different color after having been used, that those who live in a perpetual terror of fresh air might see the poisonous atmosphere to which they condemn themselves ; for all the tasteful ruralities of life are destroyed by those who dread the gentlest zephyrs, and some of our friends, even if they lived in a bottle, would wish to put the cork in."—[*Scotland and the Scotch, by Catharine Sinclair.*]

ical error in education are to be found in many boarding-schools, whose managers profess the most enlightened
views on the intellectual and physical training of youth,
and pledge themselves to the *"most scrupulous attention"*
to the health and personal comfort of their pupils.
Passing by the evils of the atmosphere of the school-
room, how often may we observe the pernicious practice
indulged in, by children, of sleeping with their heads entirely covered with the bedclothes — a habit which is often
connived at by those having the immediate charge of
their dormitories, and which seldom engages the attention, or meets with the disapprobation, of their teachers.
An occasional visit to the dormitory by the teacher, ought
to suggest many subjects of useful instruction in the
schoolroom, and no lesson can be of graver importance
to the pupil, than one in which he is taught how to preserve his own life and morals, and those of others. In
New York, and in many other parts of the Union, the
scales are at last beginning to fall from the eyes of parents, teachers, and guardians; at last, though by slow
degrees, they are beginning to appreciate the fact, and
recognise the principle, that the health and happiness of
after-life materially hinge upon the habits of children
while in their sleeping-apartments; and that (to the
credit of the managers be it told) the habit at present
under discussion has been utterly proscribed and ban-
ished from the dormitories of some of our most extensive seminaries.

Even when bedrooms are well ventilated, the breathing of good air may not be secured, on account
of the curtains, which are often drawn closely around
the bed. However fashion may sanction this custom,
it is certainly a very unwholesome one, as the air inhaled
during sleep is necessarily confined and vitiated. Those
who have entirely discarded the use of curtains expe-

rience no inconvenience, but a decided improvement in health, by the change.

By reverting to the original principles laid down in the early part of this treatise, it will be seen that besides the *pulmonary*, there is also a *cutaneous* respiration. It has been calculated that an ordinary-sized man gives off from his lungs, or rather out of his system through his lungs, about fifteen cubic feet of carbonic acid in twenty-four hours, and by cutaneous exhalation, from three to five cubic feet of the same gas, both exhalations being required to preserve the body in a healthy condition. Now let us suppose the case of a boy wrapped up in blankets, &c., with his face and head *uncovered*, but the blankets drawn so tight about his neck, that the carbonic acid from his skin will have no means of escape, and be completely imprisoned under the coverings, and also assume that three cubic feet of carbonic acid be given off from the skin in twenty-four hours, which is rather a moderate calculation; we must suppose that in a few minutes as much carbonic acid would be exhaled, as would form a stratum enclosing his whole body. The perspiration is also much increased, and bathes the body in a fluid which has a strong tendency to rapid decomposition. Thus, not only is the exhalation of carbon — a substance highly deleterious to the body, whether it be retained, or re-inhaled — absolutely obstructed by this stratum, but by an unnecessary increase of sensible perspiration, a debilitating drain is kept up on the serum of the blood, and *idio miasm* generated, which, in small quantities, has been shown to produce so many diseases, and in concentrated doses, is the virus of typhus fever.

But this is not a tithing of the evil if the head also is shrouded in, and the whole body, as it were, hermetically sealed in blankets. After the head is covered, the accumulation of carbonic acid, and of course, its peculiar effects, will increase with the time in more than a geometrical ratio. The body, narcotised and (instead of being wrapped in the sweet oblivious sleep of a well-ventilated apartment, in which no bad habits are permitted) plunged into a Lethean slumber, will occasionally throw off for a few seconds, by a kind of feverish instinct, its manifold coverings, which, no doubt, gives relief for the moment; but soon the habit is established, the body grows chilly, and the coverings are replaced. Without any stretch of imagination whatever, we must infer that a habit of this kind persisted in, especially under other circumstances unfavorable to health, for any considerable length of time, will always, and through life, influence the state of health, both corporeal and mental, and very often end in the development of scrofula, consumption, epilepsy, hydrocephaloid deformities, and possibly imbecility or idiocy.

These remarks apply at least with equal force, to the nursery. A fond, though incautious, mother or nurse, may possibly clasp her child to an affectionate bosom, while she is, in effect, administering to it slowly-operating doses of carbonic acid, and the assertion may be fearlessly hazarded, that almost as many children have been poisoned in this way as have been really *overlaid.*

On page 87 was given an account of one of those frightful results of the total neglect of providing ventilating arrangements in passenger-vessels, which appal the public mind, and for a time seem to rouse attention to the means necessary to prevent a repetition of them, little thinking, at the time of its publication in this work, that, half a century later, when knowledge and practical experience would be supposed to have made so much advance as to render the occurrence of a similar scene impossible, we should be called upon to record another, if possible still more culpable and disastrous.

It is recorded here, that it may be "kept before the people" and to show that with all the glory of its 19th century, the world, in its most civilized portions, is in disgraceful subjugation to ignorance and disregard of humanity.

The steamer Londonderry, Captain Johnston, left Sligo, at four o'clock on Friday evening, December 22, 1848, for Liverpool, with about one hundred and ninety steerage passengers — emigrants — on their way, via Liverpool, to America, and two or three cabin passengers. As she proceeded on her voyage, the weather became exceedingly foul, and after midnight, the wind rose to a perfect gale. About one o'clock that night, or rather Sunday morning, it was deemed expedient to put the steerage passengers below, and the order was executed, not, we understand, without some resistance on the part of many of them.

Most of our readers are probably acquainted with the dimensions of a steerage cabin of an ordinary steamer — a compartment rarely more than eighteen feet long, by ten or twelve in width, and in height about seven feet. Into this space, ventilated only by one opening, the companion, one hundred and fifty human beings, as we have been informed, were packed together. The steerage being thus occupied, it was next, as alleged, feared lest the water should get admission through the companion, and this — the only vent by which air could be admitted to the sufferers below — was closed, and a tarpaulin nailed over it, thus hermetically sealing the aperture, and preventing the possibility of any renewal of the exhausted atmosphere.

The steamer went on her way, gallantly braving the winds and waves, unconscious of the awful work which death was meanwhile doing within her. In the darkness and heat and loathsomeness of their airless prison, its

15

wretched inmates shrieked for aid ; and there were none to hear their cries amid the boisterousness of the storm, or if they were heard, none sagacious enough to interpret the dreadful meaning they meant to convey. At length, one man — the last, it is said, who had been put down, contrived to effect an opening through the tarpaulin of the companion, and pushing himself out, communicated to the mate that the people in the steerage were dying for the want of air. The mate instantly become alarmed, and obtaining a lantern, went down to render assistance. Such, however, was the foul state of the air in the cabin, that the light was immediately extinguished. A second was obtained, and it too was extinguished.

At length the tarpaulin was completely removed, and a free access of air admitted. When the crew went below, they were appalled by the discovery that the floor was covered by dead bodies to the depth of some feet. Men, women, and children, were huddled together, blackened with suffocation, distorted by convulsion, bruised and bleeding from the desperate struggle for existence which preceded the moment when exhausted nature resigned the strife. After some time the living were separated from the dead, and it was then found that the latter amounted to nearly one half of the entire number. Seventy-two dead bodies of men, women, and children, lay piled indiscriminately over each other, four deep, all presenting the ghastly appearance of persons who had died in the agonies of suffocation. Very many of them were covered with blood, which had gushed from the mouth and nose, or had flowed from wounds inflicted by the trampling of nail-studded brogans, and by the frantic violence of those who struggled for escape. It was evident that, in the struggle, the poor creatures had torn the clothes off each other's backs, and even the flesh from each other's limbs. Nearly all of the steerage passengers were poor farmers from the neighborhood of Sligo and Ballina, with their families, and many of the dead were naked from poverty.

An inquest was held on one of the bodies, and the jury returned the following verdict :—

" We find that death was caused by suffocation, in consequence of the gross negligence and total want of the usual and necessary caution on the part of the captain, Alexander Johnston, Richard Hughes, first mate, and Ninian Crawford, second mate ; and we therefore find them guilty of manslaughter ; and we further consider it our duty to express, in the strongest terms, our abhorrence of the inhuman conduct of the remainder of the seamen on board on the melancholy occasion, and the jury beg to call the attention of proprietors of steamboats to the urgent necessity of introducing some more effectual mode of ventilation in the steerage, and also affording better accommodations to the poorer class of passengers."*

* Belfast News Letter.

CHAPTER XV.

USE AND ABUSE OF CITIES.

First Impressions of New York upon a Stranger.—Contrast with other Cities.—Its Comparative rate of Mortality.—Impure Air may coexist with Natural Sanitary Advantages.—Foresight of its Founders.—Its High Temperature ; its Effects.—Number of Garrets and Cellars.—Basement Schools, Public School Society.—Cesspools and Privies, their great Number.—Imagination necessary to discover Realities.—The Remedy.—A new Society needed.—Particular Localities.—Five Points.—Pearl Street.—" Old Brewery." — Rag-Pickers. — Slaughterhouses. — Disadvantages of the " Croton."—The Remedy therefor.

GREAT cities have been denounced by some as great evils, and Cobbett alludes to London as a *wen*, or unnatural excrescence, growing on the body of England. They have also their advocates, who look upon them as so many centres of circulation, or foci that radiate riches, strength, intelligence, civilization, and as it were new life, to the surrounding countries. This controversy resolves itself into a question of use and abuse. There is really no well-grounded objection to great cities. They *are*, it must be acknowledged, great evils, but they are not necessarily so. All objections that have been taken to them, are founded on the erroneous structure of society inhabiting them, and the still more erroneously-constructed streets and houses in which their inhabitants live, the want of a due regard for the preservation of health, and the absence of efficient sanitary laws, to counteract the admitted increased tendency they have, to deteriorate the general health and morals. All these evils can and will be remedied. The first blows have already been struck in this peaceful campaign of benevolence, and the question is now, who are the individuals, who are the nations, to follow them up ? — Is America ? is New York to be in the front, or the rear ?

The magnitude and position of New York, being the largest city in America, justly entitle it to extraordinary consideration and justify this particular reference; and as its sanitary condition, in relation to the air breathed by its inhabitants, is very analogous to many other American cities, the succeeding remarks will generally apply to them also.

A stranger, when he first arrives in New York, is quite unprepared for the salubrity of its situation, which he soon discovers, and is disinclined to believe any longer the reports he has heard of its high rate of mortality. His mind is relieved from the narrow streets and alleys of European towns, and he is for the while led to believe, that all the streets here are Broadways and Bowerys. He no longer sees the Cimmerian fogs of London and Paris floating above his head, and occasionally descending in a darkness which can be felt; no longer the smoky canopies of Leeds, Lyons, Glasgow, or Manchester; no longer the thousands of low, and hundreds of tall chimneys, disgorging volumes of smoke and other noxious impurities; no mountain barriers to imprison the air and intercept the gentle and health-inspiring breezes; no lazy stagnant rivers to pollute the atmosphere with their pestilential effluvia; he can not reconcile his present with his past impressions; he concludes he has been misinformed. Unfortunately such was not the case. New York, with a population not one fourth that of London, and not one half that of Paris, has at least as high a rate of mortality as either of those cities, and this with

15*

a population not nearly so much condensed. Why is this? This question will be answered by a brief exposition of what is conceived to be the cause which, remotely or proximately, is most active in bringing diseases on the people and accelerating their deaths.*

The principles that have been laid down, and the facts and arguments that have been stated, imperfect though they be, afford a sufficient clue to this apparent anomaly in vital statistics, and it is easily shown that impure air may coexist with all the advantages of locality, climate, comparative exemption from smoke, and other circumstances, that deceive, not only the stranger, but also the naturalized and native citizen. Nature† has no doubt bountifully supplied the people of New York with a sufficiency of pure, wholesome air, but this avails not if they shut it out of their houses through a want of knowledge of its benefits, or be deprived of those benefits by others through ignorance, negligence, or selfishness. Their atmosphere is, to be sure, comparatively free from smoke, but there is a large amount of ingredients far more noxious substituted for it.

The streets are no doubt generally wide, and present every facility for the passage of aerial currents, but in general, the rubbish (consisting chiefly of animal and vegetable filth that is thrown upon them) is almost suffi-

---

* We are prepared to admit that, next to impure air, intemperance is the most potent agent in the increase of preventible mortality. It must be kept in mind that these two causes reciprocally produce one another. The deaths of immigrants (accelerated by foul air and other hardships on board the vessels) also enlarge the bills of mortality.

† As the word *Nature* has been occasionally employed in the course of the preceding chapters, and as "*Nature worship*" is represented to be one of the sins of the present day, it is only proper to explain, that the term has been used solely on account of its *convenience*. We have no objection to adopt the definition of Areteus, "Nature is the art of the godhead" or that of Pope :—

All are but parts of one stupendous whole,
Whose body Nature is, and God the soul."

cient of itself to inquinate those currents as effectually as any of the goitrous ravines of the Alps.

It is an historical fact that New York has attained to a greater magnitude, than any other city in the same time. Rapidity of growth is usually attended by a defective organization, and in this respect the city has both suffered and escaped. Its southern extremity will always be its nucleus, and is incapable of extension ; it was therefore fortunate, that some of the early fathers were privileged, as it were, with a glimpse into futurity, which supplied a motive for laying out its streets even so judiciously as they are. They have, by their wisdom, conferred an invaluable boon upon their posterity. Otherwise, this would have been one of the darkest plague-spots, on the face of the earth. On the other hand, there are many standing monuments of their short-sightedness, monuments quite removable, yet unremoved to the present day. If a thorough system of sewerage had been early enforced, the width of all streets regulated by law, the formation of blind lanes and alleys discountenanced, and the tenancy of cellars by human beings, either as workshops, schools, or otherwise, absolutely prohibited, a rich harvest of health and happiness, and the improved tone of morality they involve, would now be reaped, thousands of lives would have been saved or prolonged, and many hundreds of wretches, now sunk beyond reclamation, in physical and moral turpitude, would be an honor, instead of a disgrace, to the existing respectable citizens.

In estimating the influence of the different morbific agents in the city of New York, *the high temperature of the summer months must be carefully kept in view.* The thermometer very frequently fluctuates between seventy and ninety-six degrees in the shade, rising in the sun to upward of one hundred and ten degrees of Fahrinheit, for two or three months together. It is therefore clear that as the putrefaction and decomposition of animal and vegetable matter increase with the heat, the quantity of aerial poisons evolved must be much greater, and more concentrated, than in cities where the thermometer at the same season ranges between, say forty and seventy degrees. This circumstance at once accounts for the higher rate of mortality in this city, than in many others containing a larger amount of filth, and demands peculiar attention, as the same exertion in New York, might possibly remove twice as much effluvia, and of course twice as much disease, as could be done in a city of considerably lower temperature.

To put the matter in a more intelligible form, if we suppose a cart-load of offal, ordure, &c., from a slaughter-house, to give out a certain volume of fever miasm, under a temperature of sixty or seventy degrees in London; we may infer, on the principle above stated, that that volume might possibly be doubled from a similar load, under a temperature of one hundred and ten degrees in New York, Philadelphia, or New Orleans, and hence the aggravation of the evils of animal and vegetable decomposition in the warmer climates, and the greater urgency for their speedy removal.

The most deleterious atmospheric nuisances in New York, are carbonic acid, and the exhalations from animal and vegetable matter in a state of putridity. These latter consist chiefly of different combinations of hydrogen and ammonia, all of which, it is needless to repeat, are, according to the quantities contained in the air at the time of inhalation, slow or rapidly fatal poisons.[*]

As to carbonic acid, its effects are in few places felt

---

[*] In England, twenty-two children were killed by sulphuretted hydrogen, which had emanated from the contents of a cesspool. Many similar cases are on record.

with greater malignancy than in New York. There are in the city, as many as three thousand cellars, garrets, courts, alleys, and inhabited rear buildings, in which the air is to a great extent pent up, so that in calm weather it is very slowly removed, and in many cellars, garrets, and even courts, especially those forming complete *cul de sacs*, so literally hemmed in, that it remains in a state of almost complete stagnancy, for many weeks together, and these generally during the greatest heat.

Public buildings, and the first class of private houses, or stores, are in very few instances, built with a view to their complete and healthful ventilation.

Many have evidently been constructed by architects who attached due importance to strength, beauty, warmth, light, &c., but who in some unaccountable way, neglected fresh air altogether, in both ground plan and elevation.

Of the cellars or basements which are occupied by over three thousand five hundred human beings, not more than one tenth are tolerably ventilated, and many are occupied by sedentary artisans, and small grocers, who, with their wives, families, and very often a number of lodgers, live, eat, and sleep, in fact perform all their functions, in one, or at least two, small apartments. About one third of these are back basements, from which the air is still more completely excluded. The garrets, used either as daily habitations or dormitories, are at least as numerous as the basements, and are nearly as much deprived of the benefits of fresh air. These latter tenements are more generally occupied during the night, when if there chances to be a small window or two, they are scrupulously closed in winter for fear of the cold, and ignorantly or negligently allowed to remain closed in summer, thus completely excluding the outer air.

One of the worst features in the cellar habitation, is the fact that schools are still kept in them to an incredible extent, and to the incalculable deterioration of the health and morals of the children, and the unmerited discredit of the city, inasmuch as liberal means have been provided at the public expense for the efficient education of every child in it. The reason of the continuance of these schools must lie deep, and must certainly be connected with ignorance or narrowmindedness, as no sensible parent would send a child to the stupifying atmosphere of a basement, in preference to other comparatively airy apartments, where the education is greatly superior. If individuals think proper to establish schools for private instruction, they should not be discouraged, but it is only right that public disapprobation be brought to bear on those who establish them in cellars, where their intellectual faculties are as likely to be benumbed, so to speak, as their health of body is to be impaired. Children always thrive best, sleep best, and learn best, in a clear atmosphere.

The greater number of these cellar schools,* are similar in all respects to the dame-schools in Liverpool, and are kept in dwellings equally squalid and unventilated. The teachers are often old matrons, or old masters, whose systems are now antiquated, and whose attainments have not kept pace with the late rapid improvements in the profession.

These schools ought to be inspected, and reported upon by the proper authorities, who should without hesitation, suppress those kept in places unhealthy to the children. It may be objected that a number of poor people would by this means be ruined, by the loss of the only employ-

---

* It would seem that some of their teachers would object to this term as the words "*select school*" are occasionally to be observed on the shutter. This is most likely intended to anticipate any unfavorable impression.

ment by which they can support themselves. To this it may be answered that the health of the people is the first object of legislation, and that *it* ought *first* to be secured as far as possible, even though private interests should suffer, and if necessary let the state furnish other employment for those who would be thus deprived of occupation, but let not the next generation suffer for the benefit of a few of the present.

These cellar schools, however, taking the numbers they contain and the circumstances which give them origin into consideration, are innocent and tolerable, when contrasted with another class of schools, which are kept also in basements, and owe their existence, not to the destitution of the poor, the old, or the infirm, but to the patronage of the public themselves, and are superintended by a board supported by the public funds, for the express object of securing to the children of all classes a suitable education, and by which of course is understood a *healthy* education. By a reference to the "Manual of the Public School Society of the City and County of New York," for 1848, it may be seen that fourteen of their public *primary* schools are kept in basements (generally of churches) and ten in rear buildings, one of the basements being for colored children. The trustees apologise for having no primary department in Public School No. 7, on account of "*the building being without a basement ;*" implying that basement schools are fittest for very little children, and sanctioning by their high authority, the cellar schools just adverted to ; sanctioning a principle we have seen put in practice in the lowest, dampest, and worst-ventilated cellars. What motive they have in preferring a basement for the smallest of the children, it is not easy to conjecture, as a child itself might understand that its own delicate lungs and frame, are more impressible to the effects of impure air, than those of a sturdy boy or girl of twelve or thirteen.

It is most assuredly the duty of the trustees to examine these basements, and satisfy the public as well as the parents of the children, that the atmosphere of each basement is as pure and as readily ventilated as it is in the apartments where their senior classes are taught, and emancipate them from the objectionable ones before irreparable impressions are made upon their health. It is not fair that the smaller children, should be thus subjected to an invidious distinction, and be debarred the benefits of education, while their parents are paying a tax imposed for that specific object. We have heard a teacher in one of these low-ceiled basement schoolrooms, which usually contained three hundred of these little beings confined within the narrow space six hours a-day, complain severely of the sufferings she endured for want of fresh air, and this continued for months and years. She seemed aware of the cause of the evil, but the pale and puny children, had to suffer in silence and droop without relief.

Though the reader may be wearied with the frequent reference in the foregoing pages, to the great importance and general neglect of school ventilation, yet the remark may be permitted, that, with all the advancements that have been made in the art of teaching, and the great improvements which have been adopted in the internal and external arrangements of school-houses, this great and essential requisite to the perfection of both, seems yet to be very much overlooked, and too often, entirely forgotten.

Fig. 6, is a sectional view of one of the largest and most modern of the " Ward Schools" of New York, which will convey some idea of the system of *child packing*, which is followed in some of them.

The building of which this is an imperfect drawing,

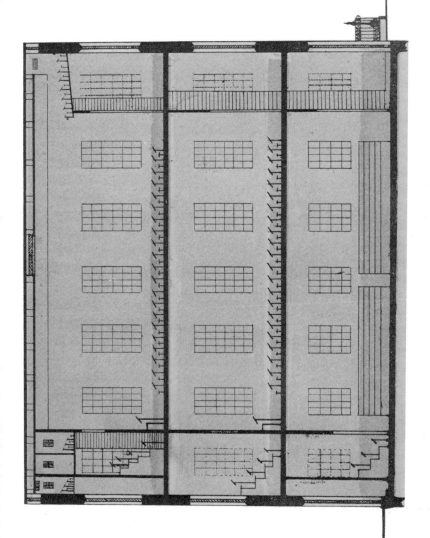

Fig. 6.

was originally intended to accommodate only 1000 pupils, but into which, 1400 have actually been suffered to be crammed, and that too, *without an attempt at systematic ventilation.*

The building is 85 feet long, by 45 feet wide, and 60 feet high from the ground to the peak of the roof, so that were there no floors, or desks, or partition walls, or pupils, or teachers, there would be about 229,500 cubic feet of air, giving for each individual 164 feet, which according to computations before given, would be reinhaled every 40 minutes, or nine times the six school-hours.

One of the objects of the Alms House in New York, is to shelter, and provide for, those unfortunate infants who are parentless, or exposed and forsaken by their unnatural mothers. Now, while there exists no question as to the general efficiency, and the spirit and motives that actuate the patrons and managers of this and some other similar charities, it is to be much regretted that the moral tendency of their benevolent exertions is far from being decided. Be this as it may, one fact can not be denied, that their objects are often frustrated by the faithlessness of the out-nurses, who are confidentially appointed, to watch over and rear these children. There is certainly no wish to bring a sweeping accusation against the nurses, thus employed, in New York, but we are warranted by authority, to state that those children will very often be found pining in dark, damp, ill-ventilated basements. A person of ordinary observation, could, from their appearance alone, determine whether they are being nursed in a basement, or high airy room. They may be known by the magnitude and unshapeliness of the head, the dilatation of the pupils of the eyes, the distorted and sunken eye-balls, the continual elevation of the hands to the face and head, as if to remove something that occasioned this

16

state of misery, the half-protruded tongue, the feeble
limbs, and in a word that general "unearthly appearance" which, in the days of superstition, used to excite
the apprehensions of the good women, that their offspring were under the influence of evil spirits; so that
there can be no doubt as to the true nature and cause of
this scrofulous and hydrocephaloid condition; which, if
not originally produced by the exclusion of fresh air,
and the other causes just specified, must undoubtedly
have been aggravated by the operation of those causes,
and now, either a fatal termination, or a useless burden
to society, during a miserable life, is almost inevitable.

If such institutions must be maintained, experience
has shown that the children ought in all cases to be taken
into, and reared in clean, well-aired hospitals, from which
noxious drugs should be carefully excluded, and the little ones kept under the eyes of those *interested* in their
moral and physical cultivation.

These facts speak volumes. To reiterate the evils
arising from this state of things, would only detract from
their magnitude, and unfit the mind to appreciate their
danger.

The emanations from animal and vegetable matter, in
a state of decomposition, operate upon the people also
as much within as out of doors. Here, as is often the
case, the greatest evils are the most hidden. It is, however, a fact ascertainable by any citizen who will make
the calculation, that there are within the municipal boundaries of the city nearly thirty thousand cloacœ; thirty thousand receptacles for large accumulations of substances,
which, of all others, are most repugnant to the senses, and
under circumstances favorable for the evolution and inhalation of their gases, the most injurious to health. To
obtain adequate impressions of the danger to which the inhabitants are exposed on this account, is absolutely impossi-

ble, as it is impossible to drag the sources of that danger to
a sufficiently clear light on paper; nor would even a bal-
loon or bird's eye view, comprehend within its circumference more than a mere segment of the ground they occupy.
Let the citizens then resort for a moment, to the fields of
imagination, and, supposing Manhattan island to be in
every respect, *except these pit-falls*, in its pristine state
of attractiveness, carry themselves back to the period of
Hendrick Hudson's first landing, and fancy what would
have been the feelings of the rude navigator and his followers, if, when walking for the first time up the island,
they had found these thirty thousand cesspools studding
it up and down, and filling the atmosphere with nauseous
gases to which their olfactories (habituated to the pure
air of the Atlantic) were strangers. Would they not
have fled the polluted shores? Would our worthy
Dutch ancestry have thought for a moment, of building
a city on a spot which, however attractive to the eye,
would prove more pestiferous than the Pontine marshes?
Yet their descendants are content to live — what brief
and sickly lives — amid the poisoned atmosphere, and
give no thought to its improvement, though so easily
accomplished.

Or, let us suppose the whole city to be at once an-
nihilated, except those nuisances. What would then
be the impressions of not only the delicate, the refined
in taste, but also of those who make no claim to nicety
of sense or sentiment? would they not also fly? To
think they would act otherwise, would be derogatory
to both taste and judgment. The sick would learn a
lesson useful if not too late, and the public authorities, so long obtuse, it is to be hoped, would at last,
after receiving no fewer than thirty thousand practical
hints on the sanitary condition of the city, come to a de-
cision, which, if acted upon, would keep at least as many

dollars a year in the pockets of its inhabitants, and confer upon them an inestimable amount of health and happiness.

These remarks are by no means strained; the objects to which they are applied, can be seen and pronounced upon at any time, and a few specimens will suffice to convince any intelligent and candid observer, that their evils are almost above exaggeration, and that until they cease to exist, the rate of mortality can never be materially diminished. The municipal authorities are certainly conducting various improvements with great energy, and on scales creditable to themselves, and lastingly beneficial to the city; but when their own and the public health are at stake, it is right that all other operations should be, if necessary, partially or wholly suspended, until the causes of disease be removed, and these thirty thousand centres of pestilence especially, no longer deal out to the lungs of the public, their noxious ex halations.

As to the practicability of preventing these accumulations, and superceding their necessity altogether by an extensive system of sewerage, analogous to that adopted in London and Paris, it is presumed no comment is necessary, since it has been demonstrated oftentimes and in many places. Why is it then that we have no laborers in this field of humanity ? Is it because such a subject may be disagreeable to discuss ? Surely not; as any person would naturally prefer to advocate this measure of cleanliness, and to remove, or pay for the removal of, these nuisances, rather than breathe over and over again for months, perhaps years, without intermission, their deleterious and offensive gases; and it should be always recollected that when the smell of any substance is perceived, the particles of that substance come in actual contact with the lining membrane of the nose, and pass into the lungs, and commingle with the blood. Is it because there is no profit connected with the work ? This can not be the case for two reasons; first, the people of New York are far from being behind in generosity, and are engaged in other works of benevolence that have no higher claims upon their liberality, without fee or reward; and secondly, it were easy to show that the measure would be a positive gain.

Is it because there is no honor or glory to be derived from the work ? No, there should be, and there are, in the city, men sufficient in number and influence, who are superior to motives so sordid; besides there are those who are fully aware, that as much glory is to be reaped in saving their own and the lives of their fellow-citizens at home, as could be gained on the plains and in the fortresses of Mexico. It might not be the effervescent glory of an Alexander, a Taylor, or a Scott, but it would be the calm, the imperishable fame of a Howard. The cause of this apathy will be left to be determined by the citizens themselves, and the suggestion be made that the grounds of their explanation will be found in the general want of information on the subject, and in the neglect of physiology and ventilation, as branches of primary instruction in schools.

" Children are the fathers and mothers of men," and on this principle what is taught children now, will be practised in the years of responsibility, when they become the heads of families, and the leaders of the community. Had the children of New York been taught the value of pure air, the necessity of ventilating their houses, and the danger of living, or attending school, in cellars, basements, and garrets, both the city and themselves would now have a different aspect. Many thousands would now breathe a pure atmosphere, who were cut off in the tender years of infancy or in ripe maturity. Late how-

16*

ever as it is, the attention of the authorities, whether legislative or municipal, should be turned to the privies. No system of cleaning (as experience has shown), except sewerage, can materially abate their effects. There will always be more than three fourths of their number in a state of constant operation, giving off their peculiar and poisonous effluvia. Cleanse them all thoroughly and at once, and like the Lernian hydra, they will immediately reappear; but let the iron be laid to the root of this most offensive and morbific of all nuisances, and it will become harmless.

New York has many noble institutions and societies, alike honorable to the nation, to the present stage of civilization, and to Christianity; but she wants one, the organization of which would confer great benefits on every inhabitant, viz.: a society analogous in its objects and principles to the " *health of towns' associations*" lately established in some parts of England. Some of the objects of such a society should be a constant surveillance, and uncompromising exposure, of the sanitary condition of all churches, schools, yards, courts, streets, lanes, workshops, &c., and investigation of the causes of the present social retrogression, of poverty and disease, and their influence on the public expenditures. Also to ascertain the vital statistics, the dimensions of apartments and houses, whose sanitary condition is suspicious, the number of inmates they contain, and above all, the loathsome *cul de sacs*, that alone degrade their inmates and disgrace the city.

Let all these be revealed to the public by accurate statistical tables, maps and descriptions, and the patrons or owners of all places prejudicial to health, remonstrated with in a friendly manner, or as the case may require, be fairly and fearlessly brought before the public by a particular reference to houses, alleys, &c., or directly by name. Such a body of individuals would no doubt have its difficulties, and its portion of slander, but these would gradually vanish as its usefulness would be developed, and its efforts begin to tell upon the population. It should do justice to every place and person, from the grandest church in the city, to the lowest purlieu in "the sixth ward." Except among the most degraded, those irretrievably lost to a sense of shame, there is still a spark left to excite improvement. Though they might prefer the endurance of the diseases induced by an impure atmosphere, and personal filthiness, to what they might call the drudgery of cleanliness, or the discomfort of cold draughts, they would make great sacrifices before they should be exposed in *print*. Next to physiological education, *exposure* will be found to be the most powerful engine that can be employed by sanitary reformers, especially to bring the lessees of such places as the Orange, Cross, and Bayard street dens of pestilence, to a sense of their duty to their fellow-mortals and themselves. From such men as these, such an association would have nothing to fear, as men without principle must also be without moral or social influence; besides, the supreme object being to consult the safety of the people, they would be effectually sheltered from vulgar imputations. The fearless exposures of Howard, Parent-Duchatelet, Chadwick, Lord Morpeth, and the different sanitary commissions that have been appointed by various governments, have probably done as much for the public health, as one half the medicine that has been swallowed since the days of the first mentioned philanthropist. Would not a like influence have like effects on this side of the Atlantic?

To enter into minute details of the various localities distinguished for their fertility in disease, and its attendant evils, would be somewhat out of place here, and from their extent impossible in such a sketch. They ex-

ist in all parts of the city.   At its very maritime thresh-
old, the state of the air is rendered very disagreeable
and unwholesome, from the manner in which some of the
quays and slips are kept.   This evil will not, however,
be entirely remedied, until the street manure ceases to
be deposited and shipped as at present.

The city authorities after having understood the necessity of a constant circulation of air in every street and
place where there are dwellers, can not but condemn
such narrow thoroughfares as Hague street and those
in its neighborhood.   In such places the air is always, in
calm weather, in a state of stagnancy.   These lanes, are,
however, comparatively healthful, when considered in
connexion with the narrow filthy alleys and *cul de sacs*,
off some of the principal streets in the city.   Many persons have, indeed, walked through the city a lifetime,
without being aware that such places exist at all.   These
must, however, look beyond plaster-of-Paris and beautiful brick facings.   To obtain a correct notion of the
swarms of human beings that, cony-like, have taken up
their abodes in holes of the earth, or congregate in garrets, they must muster the fortitude necessary to wend
their dreary and perhaps dangerous way up some filthy,
dark, winding stair, or, mole-like, burrow through the
mazy and gloomy hall of a group of cellars, all the while
stumbling over chairs and children, and wading through
broken crockery ware, vegetable refuse, and unmention-
able filth.   They must trace the monster to his den, the
last enemy of the human race to his hiding-places.   They
must explore even the "*Five-Points*" itself, that profound-
est of all sinks of moral and physical pollution, which
sends forth from its pandemonium in the shape of the
"*old Brewery*" (which is a moral brewery still) the
agents who perpetrate the "stratagems and spoils" there

concocted, and bespatter the reputation of the whole city in the eyes of the world.

A few specimens of these places would perhaps throw considerable light on them all. For this purpose, let any one (particularly if skeptical as to the alleged evils of impure air), visit some of the courts opening into the "Five-Points" or even into that great and wealthy mart, Pearl street. We shall give him two, entered at random, by a person interested in such examinations, and which are in a sanitary condition less objectionable than many others in the same quarter, viz.: those adjoining 476 and 496 Pearl street. The entrances are of considerable length, scarcely admit two persons together, and terminate in areas containing one or more privies, which occupy the centre, and are but a few feet from the doors of the houses, and of course immediately below the windows. In each case they must be resorted to by several hundreds of people. At the entrances, a stench insufferable to all except those habituated to it, meets the visiter; this increases in intensity until the inner area is arrived at, when from the height of the surrounding houses, and the consequent accumulation of the rays of the sun, very often nearly vertical, and almost torrid, he may well imagine himself in the funnel of a great chimney shaft, erected for the purpose of carrying off immense volumes of the most noxious gases, not set free by artificial lamp or fire, but by the sun itself.

The appearance of the people and their houses (if they all deserve that name), are in good keeping with the condition of the atmosphere. The doors and windows of their squalid apartments are closed against the foulness of the external atmosphere, until it is made worse within, when they are thrown open to let the still fouler air out.

Thus the inmates live from week to week, and thus

they die of fever, scrofula, debility, marasmus, and many complaints unknown to the better aired and housed. These are true specimens, of which there are endless modifications in every ward within the municipal boundaries, but especially in the locality of the Five-Points, and extending along Cross, Orange, Bayard, and Mulberry streets.

Perhaps no object in New York has proved more interesting to both stranger and citizen, than this said " old Brewery" or " distillery" or whatever it may have been intended for. It would seem as if Satan had decided that the speculation of brewing or distilling, though generally very profitable to him, was far inferior in this respect to another higher game which could be easily put in operation, and that altering his original intention, the building was fitted up for dwellers, divided into as many compartments as possible, and let to those whose finances, inclinations, or avocations, the building peculiarly suited. Along each side of the building a narrow alley* runs from Cross street, terminating in small courts in the rear. Additional doors have been broken out into the alleys, and a peep into one or two would convince the most resolute that he was in no small danger, not only of losing his health, but also of personal violence, if he has already escaped. The census of this model school of mysteries, miseries, and vice, is rated to be at times 300, that number having, it is said, actually been counted in it. In any and every aspect this is a most disgraceful spot, and contrasts very strongly, and seems strikingly inconsistent, with our boasted *model republic*, which has no doubt been often alluded to as such by many a mayor and alderman, who may have walked past the Five-Points without the *Brewery* ever once

---

* One of them, is usually called " Murdering Alley."

catching their eye, or suggesting any thought of improvement, which should long ago have been enforced.

As to the number of rooms in the Brewery we have no means of ascertaining it, but its low situation and its external appearance with the number of occupants compared with its size, speak loudly enough for its state of ventilation. There seems only to be one privy which occupies the centre of the small area of the court, but of its state, and the condition of the atmosphere around it, for a considerable distance, the reader will have no objection to waive a description. It would seem that the influence of habit, and the self-fortifying principle, inherent in the human constitution, in a great measure, shields those miserable and degraded wretches, who inhabit such places, from immediate dissolution, while the pestiferous atmosphere gradually extinguishes all the better attributes of their nature.*

There are however, about the Five-Points, and indeed many other parts of the city, equally as great eye-sores to all interested in the advancement of society, as the house referred to, except perhaps in the particular of absolute population. In the lower part of Washington street, and in the narrow streets and lanes in its vicinity, there are during the emigration season, many suitable counterparts to the house in Boston. As many as two dozen of the adventurers often sleep in an apartment not more than twenty-four feet square, the air being in a worse state if possible than in the ships. From these houses many emerge, as paupers, their pockets emptied,

---

* The following paragraph is quoted from the "Boston Bee": "*Life in Boston.*—There is in Oliver street, a house containing thirteen rooms which has for regular occupants *ninety-three persons.*" A New York editor adds, "'The *Old Brewery,* new edition;' but it has been seen that the Boston establishment is still deep in the shade of our old Brewery. Yet, who would have imagined, that lodgings would ever be so dear and mortals so extravagantly gregarious in this land of bricks and timber."

and their bodies debilitated, unable to work, and often
even unable to beg.

Another source of atmospheric impurity in the city is
the notorious trade of rag-picking. Of the impropriety
of permitting this occupation to be carried on in its present unrestricted way, there can not be two opinions. The
fact is repeatedly alluded to by the authorities and corroborated by daily observation, that scarcely anything
tends more to pollute the air, than the accumulations of
old rags imbued with every species of filth, and covered
with vermin. They constitute the lurking-places of
those contagious fevers that occasionally devastate the
neighborhoods in which the houses for these *wares* are
kept. This is the concurrent testimony of all sensible
persons living near such places. A statistical return of
these places, and their lessees would be, for reasons already alluded to, particularly valuable.

Slaughterhouses are the next most conspicuous nui-
sance, and are not much less injurious to health. It is
agreed, in all places where their effects are investigated,
that they ought to be excluded from all great cities.
New York can be supplied with an abundance of fresh
vegetable productions from the country, why not with
meat also? For such facilities as these, perhaps no other
city is so favorably situated ; and it is to be hoped the
day will shortly arrive, when its citizens will know, and
not be afraid to do their duty, and appoint men to direct
their municipal affairs who will adopt all just and legal
means to protect the public health, in this and all other
matters.

If we ascend from the purlieus of the Five-Points
and Orange street, the lowest boarding-houses and the
rag-stores and shambles, to hotels and steamboats, some
of them of the first standing, we find the air inhaled by
their lodgers and passengers improves much less, than,

from the external appearance of the latter, would have been expected. We find that these stately fabrics have seldom or never any systematic ventilation, their saloons and chambers being in almost every instance, defective in any efficient means for drawing off the foul air. The oyster-saloons are no less defective; many of them have only one opening, by which the air is to pass both out and in. Such places are not likely to keep up either a good appetite, or good nature, and most certainly they are often visited without refreshment or exhilaration. The river-steamers, those "floating palaces," cry still louder for reform, and surely the government which has enacted so many good laws for the protection of travellers and immigrants, might with equal propriety enforce proper sanitary measures in these vessels also. The immigrant, broken down by the inhalation of foul air in the ship coming over, and in the boarding-house, pays his passage up the river *including a berth;* but he soon finds, after he has taken up his quarters for the night, that he must choose between two things: to remain and be suffocated or poisoned in a crowded cabin, or pass the night on deck in the open air. Possibly many have lost their lives from the effects of impure air, or exposure during the night, in these "*whited sepulchres.*"

The Croton water, though it has conferred invaluable benefits on the people of New York, has, under existing circumstances, been also a source of many pressing, but remediable disadvantages. The pumps that were going in all parts of the city, formerly drained the subsoil to a very considerable extent; but now, since they have been abandoned, the water percolates into the substratum and into the floors of the cellars, which become saturated; and the fact that many basements have become *untenantable,* is proof positive that vast numbers of families who must choose between living in such places, and

17

living in the street, are wretched in the extreme, from a
floor constantly wet and the air loaded with moisture, in
addition to its other impurities.

The putrefaction of garbage, and of every species of
vegetable and animal filth, which imperfectly operative
laws still permit to be thrown on the streets, is greatly
facilitated by their constant saturation with the water
from the private houses, and hence the effluvia from the
stagnant water in the subsoil, and from street dirt (considerably increased by the pigs, which seem to enjoy
more immunities and privileges in this city than any of
the other lower animals), have much increased since the
introduction of the water.

How easy it is for the citizens to understand, that the
soil on which the city is built should have been first prepared for this magnificent and useful undertaking. But
yet it is not too late. Let them next agitate for an extensive and efficient system of sewerage, to drain off the
water after its benefits have been made available, and
with it, if possible, all the garbage, refuse contents of
sinks, privies, &c., into what has been ingeniously and
happily termed the " great wash tub of the Atlantic."
Measures of waterage, drainage, and ventilation, ought
in all cases to be concurrent.

It has been calculated that in London, 60 tons of carbonic acid, and 60 tons of water, are given off from the
lungs of human beings in one day! Of these, large
quantities must be reinhaled. Assuming the population
of New York to be nearly one fourth that of London,
and including the animals, there can not be much less
than 20 tons of each daily exhaled. From the narrow-
ness of the streets, and the defective ventilation of the
houses, dilution by pure air is impeded, and reinhalation
is the necessary result. After describing the well-like
courts and alleys of Liverpool, in connexion with this

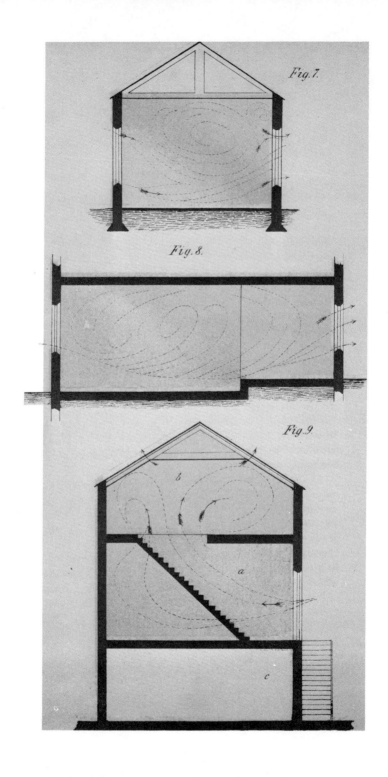

Fig.7.

Fig.8.

Fig.9.

part of the subject, Dr. Duncan says he hails with delight the approach of a hurricane or thunder-storm. There is no doubt that these have often been to the people of New York, blessings in disguise.

These few suggestions have been offered with the belief, that, if they be acted upon by the citizens themselves and those they appoint to make their laws, New York will become, what she ought to be and can be, one of the most healthful cities in the world.

The present chapter may be appropriately closed by presenting drawings of the manner in which the foul air of many school-houses, churches, &c., accumulates in some parts more than others, according to the direction of the wind and other causes, and which are supposed generally, but very erroneously, to be ventilated by the windows. The space colored *red*, represents the extent and amount of the pure air, under the most favorable circumstances of a strong wind, and the *blue* space indicates the extent and degree of impure atmosphere.

Fig. 7 is an illustration of the usual progress of air in a school, church, or lecture-room, when occupied, and ventilated by windows, the fresh air predominating on one side, and the vitiated air at the other.

Fig. 8 illustrates the progress of air in a large school, where, when the wind inclined in the direction indicated, the junior pupils, seated on an elevated platform, were exposed to a highly-vitiated atmosphere. This is the arrangement of many of the public schools of New York.

Fig. 9 is an illustration of the state of the air in a school-house, in which the vitiated air from the lower room (*a*) affords the only supply to the upper room (*b*). This state of things is pre-eminently marked in the uppermost apartments and gallery of the house, represented in fig. 6. The only air for the 100 children in the attic-rooms is supplied from the lungs of the 400 a few feet below them.

CHAPTER XVI.

Observations on Practical Ventilation; Notice of some of the popular Errors
on the Subject.

It is not more important to understand the necessity
of breathing pure air, than to know the proper means
necessary, under various circumstances, to realize its
benefits.   A person may build a house, while at the laying of each brick he is impressed with all the facts and
arguments that have been employed in the foregoing
pages, and yet fail to supply the apartments with a sufficiency of fresh air.   In fact, few parts of their art appear less understood by builders and architects than
that of warming and ventilating at the same time; and it
is very seldom that pure and artificially warm air are
breathed together.   This is owing, in a great measure, to
many popular errors that exist in reference to the nature, properties, and effects, of heat, and the laws which
govern the currents of the atmosphere, and regulate the
diffusion of gases.

The first principle to be observed in relation to the
means to be put in practice for ventilating rooms or
buildings, is that of the *agitation* of the air itself; for it
is by this only that the atmosphere can be thoroughly
renovated.   As has been happily expressed by Cowper,
in his poem of " The Sofa"—

> * * * "By ceaseless action all that is subsists.
> Constant rotation of the unwearied wheel
> That Nature rides upon, maintains her health,
> Her beauty, her fertility.   She dreads
> An instant's pause, and lives but while she moves.

Its own revolvency upholds the world.
Winds from all quarters agitate the air,
And fit the limpid element for use,
Else noxious. Oceans, rivers, lakes, and streams,
All feel the freshening impulse, and are cleansed
By restless undulation."

The same principle which is thus expressed as applicable on the scale of the whole atmosphere agitated by winds, applies with greater force to those comparatively *atomic* portions embraced within the narrow confines of the walls of buildings; and a quiescent atmosphere, unrenewed by either natural or artificial currents, is very soon found to be oppressive and disagreeable.

In pointing out the means of practical ventilation, adapted to the great majority of dwellings, workshops, churches, schoolhouses, &c., the first axiom to be remembered is, that

Purity of the atmosphere can not be maintained without its being disturbed by currents, which cause its different parts to be continually changing places.—As this is the first law to be regarded in relation to the subject of ventilation, happily the nature of the aerial fluid is such that not only is it very easy to produce the necessary motions in the air, but it would be very difficult entirely to prevent them.

The *natural* causes which principally produce aerial movements are, 1st, changes of temperature; and 2d, intermixture of the different gases which enter the air from various sources.

The atmosphere possesses greater mobility than any other natural substance. The slightest variations of temperature, even such as are entirely inappreciable by our senses, cause expansion or condensation in some part of the mass affected, and changes of place in those parts necessarily ensue.

Heat expands the air, that is, makes it thinner, and

17*

therefore lighter; hence it rises, and the colder air in the neighborhood being heavier, rushes in to supply its place, and keep up an equilibrium. This fact is illustrated by every fire that burns, whether it be a taper, or the conflagration of a city. A light flock of cotton held over a candle will be carried upward by the gentle current produced by the flame, and the huge masses of burning wood which are often driven hundreds of feet, testify the strength of the blast caused by the burning houses.

On the other hand, cold condenses the air, and its tendency is then downward to a place where its density is less. Thus are produced every variety of aerial movement, from the hurricane to the gentle breeze.

The air in houses is affected in the same way, but on a smaller scale, by fires or natural animal heat, which raise the temperature, and of course rarefy the air; while, on the contrary, the walls, windows, &c., by absorbing the heat, diminish the temperature, and thus numerous small currents are continually setting from the densest portions of the air to the most rarefied; or in other words from the coldest to the hottest. The heat of the sun, as it increases toward noon, and diminishes at evening, produces the same effects on a larger scale.

Where two bodies of air of different temperatures are placed near each other, and communicate by small apertures, an intermixture of the two will go on more or less rapidly, by currents passing between them. This is exemplified by the warm air of a parlor, and the cold air of a hall, mixing with each other by a double current, where the door which separates them is opened a short distance. A candle held near the top of the door will show a current of warm air passing *out* of the room, and a candle near the floor will show a current of cold air flowing *into* the room. (See fig. 10.) These

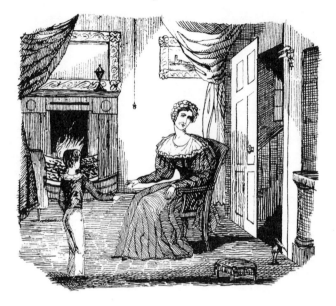

Fig. 10.

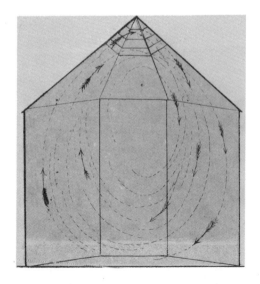

Fig. 11.

currents will continue until the two bodies of air arrive at an equality of temperature.

In like manner, the cold air of a dirty street or filthy court, impregnated with noxious effluvia, is continually rolling into the adjacent cellars, while the air in those habitations, made warm by respiration and combustion, makes its exit at the top of the door.

The same phenomenon is observed when different parts of the same body of air, are subjected to changes of temperature, as in large apartments which have a sky-light or a thin roof over them. The warm air, as it rises and impresses against the sky-light or roof, gives its caloric to the latter, becomes denser, and accordingly falls, thus causing regular currents *upward* on one side of the room, and *downward* on the other side. This is represented in fig. 11. The cold glass of a common window will produce a similar effect, as is noticed on another page. Thus also when a fire is built below the tall column of air in a chimney it soon heats and rarefies that column, which rises and forms a partial vacuum to fill up which the colder air near the floor of the room rises, leaving, in turn, a partial vacuum in its place, to supply which, air from without flows in through the windows and doors, and thus a *draught* is established, which less or more perfectly carries off both the air of the room, and the smoke.

There is also another species of movement going on among the gases composing the air, not less important, though not so observable.—It is found, by experiment, that the specific gravity of nitrogen, one principal ingredient of the air, is less than that of oxygen, the other ingredient, and that of carbonic acid much greater than either. From this it might be inferred, especially as they are not chemically, but mechanically, combined, that they would enclose the globe in three strata, like the coats of an onion, nitrogen being uppermost, oxygen next, and carbonic acid nearest the surface. This, however, is not the case; and if this arrangement should exist for only a few minutes, every animal would be poisoned and destroyed. These gases are found in almost exactly the same proportion, in the densest and the most rarefied volumes of atmosphere, on the tops of the highest mountains and in the bottoms of the lowest valleys, in town and in country, except there is some accidental obstruction to their proper combination, such as in certain mountain gorges, very narrow streets, mines, caves, houses (especially basements), ships, &c., where oxygen is exhausted faster than it can be supplied by the adjacent air, and carbonic acid evolved faster than it can be carried off.

The physical law which effects this equal mixture, or, as it is called, "mutual diffusion of gases," has been lately fully investigated, and is no less simple and beautiful than important. Mr. Dalton ascertained that *each gas was a vacuum for another*, and that all gases are capable of absorbing one another, thus making an equal mixture. For example: he put carbonic acid into a cylinder below another cylinder containing hydrogen, a gas twenty times lighter, and found, after some time, they had formed a perfectly homogeneous mixture in both vessels — the carbonic acid rising in opposition to the laws of gravity, and the hydrogen descending.

This occurs much in the same way that water is taken up by evaporation, or as salt, when put into a full glass of water, mixes with it. The salt and water are both porous, and consist of particles; the particles of the water having a greater attraction for the salt than they have for one another, and so with those of the salt with respect to the particles of water. The consequence is, that the interstices among the particles of one substance are filled up by the particles of the other, and the glass does not run over.

In like manner, a quantity of carbonic acid will, if unimpeded, fill up the interstices in a quantity of oxygen, and become equally mixed with it, without reference to specific gravity. In both cases there is a considerable obstruction offered by the particles, and therefore the combination is not *instantaneous* but *gradual*. Thus is briefly explained the second general cause of aerial currents.

It will now appear little wonderful that man, who has chosen to live within walls, and in situations where the operation of this law is impeded, has suffered so much from its almost uniform infringement, and still less that the savage who prefers the wilderness, has infinitely better health.

Some of the prevailing errors growing out of the non-observance of the simple principles just laid down, require particular notice. *The primitive error seems to consist in ignorance of the constituents of the air, and in the idea that it is a simple substance.* The fact that a person could possibly live a short time in almost any quality of air, without any suddenly-developed effects, discouraged inquiry into the matter, and disarmed the terrors of atmospheric impurities to a considerable extent. People therefore built their houses and towns without reflecting on the subject; and the accidental apertures and crevices kept up the delusion, by giving them in all cases a supply, though a scanty one. In more enlightened ages they seem to have admitted the necessity of fresh air, but considered its removal as very rapid and very easily accomplished. This, as has been explained, is not the fact.

To effect a speedy removal of vitiated air, there must be in all cases a very free communication between it and the pure air. Hence the unwholesomeness of a small room, with several occupants, in winter, with the windows and doors shut as close as possible — heated by a stove — with no renewal of air, except by the small quantity that oozes slowly through the crevices. There are many cases of this kind, in which not a suspicion arises among the inmates of the deficiency and impurity of the air they are breathing. The fire, indeed, rarifies the air in the chimney, which produces a draught, but only from the part adjacent to the floor. A supply of fresh air to the lungs, therefore, is impossible, in quantities sufficiently vitalizing, and the penalty of ignorance and neglect will surely be inflicted. To throw the door of a room open in these cases improves the state of the air a little; but the air in the hall will, perhaps, soon become exhausted, and the condition of the air breathed will not be materially altered. Suppose the door thrown open to the external air, or another chamber receiving a constant supply, then the air may become respirable and tolerably pure while the fire continues; but when the fire is burned out, or, as in summer, altogether absent, no sufficient ventilation can be kept up in the room by the door alone, as now the draught in the chimney has ceased. The carbonic acid, and the different animal exhalations, will accumulate to a certain extent in the room, — or, in other words, will not be interchanged with the pure gases outside the door as quickly as they are produced. The windows must then be depended upon, which, however, on account of the weather, can not perhaps be opened — and even when opened, there can not always be produced a sufficiently rapid diffusion of the gases to avoid the evils of the impure air.

Nor must it be forgotten, that the renewal of the air by an ordinary fireplace, is mostly of that part only

Fig. 12.

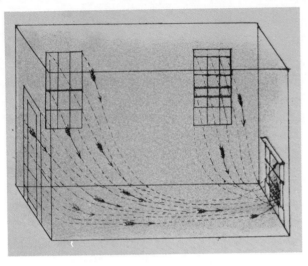

Fig. 13.

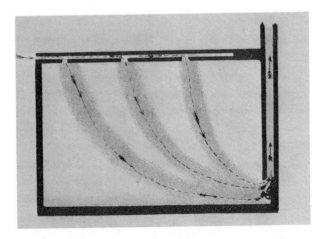

which is near the floor. The mouth of the chimney is generally below the heads of the inmates, and the impure air of the room, being warmest, is lighter and rests uppermost; and the cooler and heavier air, which is lowest, is the only part of the atmosphere of the room which is sufficiently renewed;—that portion in which the head is immersed, remains more or less unrenewed and liable to be reinhaled: that which enters through the crevices of the doors and windows into a warm room, on a cold day, falls more or less suddenly to the floor, and moves toward the fireplace (see fig. 12), up which it ascends, leaving the rest of the area of the room with its atmosphere unrenewed. The practice has sometimes been adopted of causing a current of air, properly warmed, to flow into a room through apertures in the ceiling; the draught caused by the fire would aid its passage downward, and remove it as fast as it reached the floor, thus producing a change in the entire atmosphere of the room, as illustrated by fig. 13.

This shows, to some extent, the difficulty of warming and ventilating simultaneously, and that some other means than those that are accidental in the building of the house must be resorted to.

One of the commonest misconceptions connected with this subject, is, that when persons sit with their backs to the window, they are liable to take cold, from the cold air penetrating through the panes or crevices of the window.

This is very often supposed to be the case when there is, in reality, no current of air setting through the crevices; but the true explanation is, in many instances, that the glass, cooled by the cold air outside, abstracts the heat from the air inside, or, in other words, cools it down; and as it is now heavier than the surrounding air, or that in the middle of the room, a downward current is produced. If in very cold weather, when a room is heated, a candle be held opposite one of the panes of a window, or below a skylight, the flame will be carried downward, without any air entering from without. But the heat from the person himself will also be conducted off by the cold window, and the *sensation*, as of a current of cold air, will be felt, when there will be none in reality. Those who believe, therefore, that a room is sufficiently ventilated by common windows, and find proof in these alleged currents, by trying the experiment above mentioned, will perceive their error.

This inconvenience is avoided by double windows with a stratum of air between, though then at the expense of what little fresh air does sometimes come in through the crevices. The stratum of air thus confined prevents, almost altogether, the transmission of heat either outward or inward, and this principle has been successfully applied in the construction of ice-houses. When the temperature of the air in the room is equal to that of the air outside, there is evidently no more danger of catching cold at the window than in any other part of the room.

With regard to chimneys, it is the common idea that the wider they are, the easier will the smoke and air make their exit. The contrary is more nearly the fact, as the column of air in the chimney, when smaller, is more rapidly heated, and the column of cold air above it, outside, diminished in its lateral section, and therefore not so heavy and obstructive. A medium diameter must be adopted to insure efficient draught and ventilation; and when other means of ventilation exist, the dimensions evidently need not exceed those of a common stove-pipe, which, when only eight or ten inches in diameter, carries off the smoke perhaps better than if eighteen or twenty.

Another error, requiring notice in this place, is a very

common one — that the carbonic acid gas eliminated from the lungs and skin, being naturally much heavier than the air, falls toward the floor, and will be found more abundant at the bottom than at the top of the room.

Were this true, the ventilation produced by a fire in a chimney, or an open stove, would be sufficient in almost any ordinary case. But such is not the fact, for two reasons: 1st, the air thrown off from the lungs is nearly at the temperature of the body itself, and is therefore *warmer*, and consequently *lighter*, than the surrounding atmosphere: on this account it rises.—2d, by the law of diffusion, just explained, all the gases found in the atmosphere are immediately and rapidly diffused among each other, unless prevented by some other law, such as temperature. Any one who tests the matter will find that the uppermost parts of a room, especially of such as are occupied by numbers of people, are almost always the most oppressive and disagreeable. This accounts for the greater unpleasantness of the galleries of a church or a theatre than the lower seats. The pressure of the warm air is *upward*, and the carbonic acid, warmed like the rest, seeks the same position rather than a lower one.

Still another very frequent error is, that a cool atmosphere is necessarily fresh or pure; and the idea is very prevalent, that by sleeping in a cool room, all the advantages of pure air are obtained. A little reflection will show, that, in this view, the *temperature* of the air is confounded with its *quality*, which have no necessary connexion whatever with each other. Nor is it any more true, as is sometimes supposed, that a *warm* atmosphere is necessarily *impure*. The quality of a gas does not depend upon its temperature; a person may breathe an impure air at any temperature, high or low, and the same with a pure air. The air of a bedroom will be-

18

come impure, if unventilated, in the coldest weather, and an atmosphere warmed either naturally or artificially may be inhaled in perfect purity, if properly ventilated.*

In the application of means for practical ventilation,— that is, for removing foul air from a room, and introducing fresh air into it,— the first thing to be considered and obtained *is a motive power*.

As has already been stated, currents are very easily established in a body of air; and variations of temperature, and the law of diffusion, are almost constantly at work, producing changes of place among the various parts of any specific portion of the atmosphere.

But it will be perceived that motions thus produced in a body of air, isolated and having no communication with the external atmosphere, can have no effect to purify it. Take, for instance, the air of a chamber occupied at night by several persons, or of a schoolroom in the daytime, whose air is inhaled by a number of pupils, and which is cut off from any communication with the external air by the windows being closed, the chimney-throat stuffed tight, and all other crevices made impervious: in either case, the heat of the bodies, and the carbonic acid and other gases eliminated from the lungs, skin, &c., will produce movements in the air of the room; but the impure air can not escape from the room, nor can the movements thus established have the effect to purify the air in any degree.

The removal of the impurities from, and the introduction of fresh air into the room, are essential to the main-

---

* When it was asserted by the keeper of a certain penitentiary establishment, not long since, that the plan of ventilation adopted by him in the institution was in all respects complete and sufficient, the air being at all times free from impurities,—and when the fact was doubted upon an examination of the plan,—he answered, that it was proved by the upper tier of cells being no *hotter* than the lower tier: thus testing the quality of the air by the *thermometer*.

tenance of a wholesome air, whether in a room of large or small dimensions. For the effectual ventilation of an apartment, there must therefore be a constant stream of air flowing in, and also a constant one flowing out. This stream, or (what is much preferable) *streams,* should not be more perceptible at one part of the room than at another, and should be duly warmed or cooled, according to the season, and the causes contributing to produce changes in its temperature,—and all this without injury to its vitalizing qualities.

The ingress of air into an apartment is called its *plenum movement*—its egress, the *vacuum movement*—and both combined, the *mixed* movement.

The windsail for ventilating ships is a familiar example of the *plenum* method, and the exhausting of the receiver of an air-pump an example of the *vacuum* movement. The draught of a chimney is also a familiar instance of the latter.

When either one or the other of these two methods is employed alone, there can be no certainty that the foul air of a room is all removed ; in other words, there is no surety that the ventilation is perfect ;—but when the two are combined, and the *mixed* method is put in operation with a proper degree of diffusion, then, as the force of the currents is proportioned to the necessities of the case, may the ventilation be said to be complete.

A motive power being necessary to a sufficiently rapid and complete removal of the foul air from an apartment, and the substitution, in its place, of a sufficient amount of pure air, it is necessary here to notice another error, which, though of less seriousness than some that have been mentioned, is as frequent as any.

It is generally supposed that a simple crevice in any part of a room — as for instance the crack of a door or window, or the aperture of a fire-flue — affords a sufficient

*opportunity for the escape of the impure, and the intro-
duction of pure air.* In many instances, where a room
is of large dimensions, and occupied by but two or three
people, it is possible that this may answer the purpose;
but when the amount of impure air generated is large,
such means are quite inadequate: for, in the first place,
the only powers to cause a change of air, in general,
are the two that have been mentioned, viz., the *difference
of temperature* and the *law of diffusion*, with neither, nor
both, of which, can the interchange be sufficiently rapid
for a small apartment. It has been already said, that
even in the open air, in a still day, a sense of oppression
may be perceived in a crowd.

The smallest aperture is, of course, better than none;
but *in the absence of any direct motive power*, no dependence can be rightly placed upon such openings. As
reasonable would it be to suppose the air in a bottle
would fly out by extracting the cork, as that the air of a
room would all escape through the crack of a door, or
the aperture of an open window.

It is necessary to notice here another error, as common, almost, as it is singular and absurd, which is generally discovered by a dialogue like the following:—

[Scene—A church, public-hall, court-room, lecture-
room, public school, or any other large apartment, with
costly fitting up, and an aperture in the ceiling, which
is a few feet below the roof.]

Enter Stranger, and sees the *Architect* inspecting the
work.

Stranger. Good morning, sir! this promises to be a
beautiful edifice when finished, evincing much taste and
liberality of means.

Architect. Glad to hear you think so; we have done
our utmost, in accordance with the true principles of
architecture, to make a handsome and convenient edifice.

Strang. Of course you have not neglected that most important matter for the comfort and health of the audience, ventilation?

Arch. By no means, as you may see by turning your eyes to the ceiling; that aperture you observe there, is to be ornamented with one of the most beautiful designs in the city.

Strang. It will, no doubt, be beautiful to the eye. But how do you expect to get rid of the foul air?

Arch. Oh! the aperture will be always open, though the holes will be concealed in the ornamental work, and through them all the bad air will go off.

Strang. What will become of it, after it has passed through those openings?

Arch. Why, then I suppose it will get out through the roof, of course.

Strang. Then, of course, you have left openings in the roof, for it to escape by?

Arch. Oh! no; that was not thought necessary, as it can get out through the cracks and crevices which are always to be found; and if there are none, it gets into the loft or attic above the ceiling, and stays there, and that is all that is required.

Strang. But when the attic is full (which will be in a few minutes, with a large audience), what will you do with the rest of the foul air which is continually thrown off from the lungs, lamps, and fires, below? How is that to escape?

Arch. Really, I can not answer you. Your question puzzles me.

Strang. But further, Mr. Architect: did it never occur to you that this opening in the ceiling is not only no relief at all, but is indeed worse than nothing?

Arch. It never did, and I think you will find it hard to prove that. It certainly gives escape to *some* of the foul air; as much as the attic will hold, at least.

18*

Strang. Not so, by any means. You admit that the foul air, which is warmest and therefore lightest, rises and passes through the opening in the ceiling into the attic; but there it comes in contact with the roof, which is much colder, and takes the surplus heat from the foul air, by which the latter is made heavier, and consequently falls back again into the room below, and descends to the lungs of the people. You will generally find a double current passing through the opening in the ceiling, one, upward, of *warm* foul air, the other downward, of the same air *cooled* (as illustrated by fig. 11).

Arch. You have indeed proved your statement, which I have never before thought of. But we can remedy the evil by putting windows in the attic, or making small openings under the eaves of the roof, through which the foul air would escape and not return.

Strang. There are several objections to that mode of relief. In the first place, if those windows you propose are not easily accessible, they would not be opened at the proper time; and even if they were accessible, their regulation must be left to a sexton or janitor, who perhaps would be entirely ignorant of the principles of aerial currents. On the other hand, both the windows and other apertures you have spoken of, if left open, would not only give exit to the warm impure air, but would also admit the cold air directly upon the heads of the audience below, which would be uncomfortable, if not insupportable and dangerous.

Arch. Now that you state the matter so clearly, I remember often to have heard complaints of cold draughts, unpleasant odors, sleepy feelings, &c., made by individuals, but have always put them down as lazy or nervous people, and attributed their discomfort to anything but what now appears to be the true cause, that is, the foul air of the church or lecture-room they were sitting in. I see that I have wholly misunderstood the subject, and would be glad to know what plan can be adopted to remove the impure air, and at the same time avoid the objections you have mentioned.

Strang. Many of the difficulties may be obviated by connecting the opening in your ceiling with a tube in the attic, which should terminate in the smoke-flue, which, being warmed in winter, would carry off some of the foul air, without admitting any cold air. A better plan would be to terminate that tube in a separate shaft projecting above the roof, and surmounted with an exhausting cowl, such as Mott's or Emerson's. These plans, however, would rectify the evils only partially, and without sufficient certainty; to ventilate *thoroughly* and *continually*, some plan for the regular admission of pure air, as well as for the removal of the impure air, must be adopted. The plans for this purpose I can not explain now, but you will find the details for them in books on the subject.

Arch. I thank you heartily for this interview, and shall at once study the subject fully.

Strang. Allow me to suggest another idea to you, which is, that when you next are employed to erect a *church* edifice, to put the *steeple* to the only real use it is capable of, and make it a means of ventilating the body of the house. Every church-steeple presents a means of ventilating unsurpassed for efficiency, and which would add little or nothing to its cost. Good-morning.

One of the simplest motive powers for ventilation, and one most readily obtained in almost every description of room or house, is *Heat*. Every fire that burns, and every flue that is warmed, are means of ventilation, more or less efficient according to the manner in which their power is put to use. No fire can burn without causing a draught of air, and no flue can be warmed without causing more or less motion in the column of air it encloses, both of which may be applied to the exhaustion of any room with which they are connected.

The fuel in a stove or grate must draw the air for its combustion from the apartment in which it is placed; the vacuum thus produced must be supplied either from the adjoining rooms, or directly from the external air, through the doors and windows, and, as far as it goes, there is *change of air* produced in the room. But under ordinary circumstances, as is shown by fig. 12, the cold air, when it enters from without, through the crevices of doors or windows, being heavier, falls more or less directly to the floor, and is not sufficiently commingled with the general atmosphere of the apartment to constitute ventilation of it.

The important fact being established, that *in every heated flue there is more or less vacuum, which will cause a current to set into it through any opening which may be made into it, to any extent until the vacuum is removed*, we have a means of ventilation of almost universal applicability, and in general sufficient for ordinary dwellings.

There are various modes in which the vacuum power of a heated flue may be employed to exhaust the foul air from a room. One mode is shown in fig. 14, in which the flue of a common fireplace is represented with an aperture cut in it near the ceiling of the room, through which, if there is sufficient draught, a current is established, which must necessarily remove the air of the room. In a chimney of sufficient height, there is generally enough draught to maintain a constant current into the flue through this opening.

This method of applying the exhausting power of a heated flue to the ventilation of a room, exhibits the principle or basis upon which a great variety of arrangements may be made, and it has at the same time the important

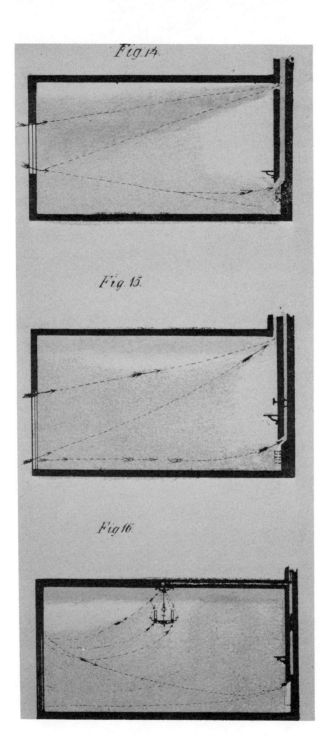

Fig. 14.

Fig. 15.

Fig. 16.

advantages of great simplicity, economy, and ease of construction. It consists of nothing more, in fact, than cutting a small hole through the brick wall of the flue, in any convenient situation in the room through which the flue passes. For the ventilation of the bedroom, or parlor of an ordinary dwelling, an aperture of five or six inches diameter will generally be ample for the removal of all the impure air, unless the number of occupants is uncommonly large. The aperture may be made by the simple removal of two or three bricks, or it may be made circular, like the opening of an ordinary stove-pipe. It may be obscured from view by suspending in front of it, at a short distance, a picture, behind which the air will pass to it, as readily as if it is left uncovered, and there are many rooms in which the opening may be cut into the flue at the side of the jamb or breastwork, so that it will be unobserved by an ordinary visiter.

It will be apparent to all, that where there are a number of fireplaces in a house, each of which must have a separate flue, there are the same number of opportunities for ventilation by this plan ; and in an ordinary two or three story dwelling-house, where there are six or eight flues, it is an easy matter to secure a ventilation for each room, to an extent sufficient for all ordinary purposes. This plan is based upon the supposition, that the draught of the chimneys is strong enough to prevent any regurgitation, by which smoke would be driven back into the room. If it is not, the draught should be increased by the application of some means to secure that end, among the easiest of which will be found that of surmounting the chimney with Mott's or Emerson's exhausting cowl, a description of the former of which will be given in another page.

The ventilating opening here described should be commanded by a valve or register, for the purpose of being closed when the fire is being kindled, or when the room requires to be heated, as not only does the air of the room escape, but a considerable portion of the heat of the apartment is carried off through it also.

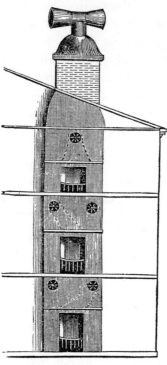

The plan here proposed, will ventilate dwellings in summer, and secure a good draught to the chimney in winter. The adjoining cut represents the chimney with the fireplaces on each floor of a three-story house. The registers on each side under the ceiling, are connected with the flues. They can be closed or opened at pleasure. By closing the grate in summer, and opening the register, the cap on the chimney will cause a constant current of pure air to flow through every room in the house. By reversing the openings, a good draught will be secured for winter. By leaving the registers open when using fires, no injurious effect can arise from gas, even in sleeping apartments. The cap figured on the chimney (the invention of J. L. Mott) is one designed to be made of cast iron. It will set over the mason-work, bind it together, protect all from the weather, secure draught and ventilation, and make a handsome finish.

A modification of this plan is exhibited in fig. 15, by which is represented a flue for ventilation only, unconnected with the smoke-flue, but built in immediate contact with it, so that it may be warmed by it. As in this arrangement the separate ventilating flue can contain no smoke or gases, no fear need be entertained of their being driven back into the apartment; but in this case the draught can not be so strong as in the other, for the reason that the flue can not receive so much heat—all that it obtains being through the brick wall which separates it from the smoke-flue. In a *stack* of chimneys, such as are found in dwellings of common construction, several of these separate ventilating flues may readily be built in between the smoke-flues, from which they would derive a temperature enabling them to act in a greater or less degree.

The principle being understood that a heated flue, or chimney, will draw into itself portions of the surrounding air with which it may be connected, it may now be readily understood how a room, at a distance from the flue, may be ventilated by *connecting the two together by a tube.* This method has been advantageously employed to ventilate the workshops of manufacturing establishments, which had on the premises tall chimneys connected with powerful fires; and it has even been applied, and very successfully, to ventilate the dwellings of the workmen in the vicinity. This is done by uniting the interior of the dwellings with the interior of the chimney-shaft: the exhausting power of the heat in the latter has been found sufficient to ventilate several tenements at once.

This mode of connecting a room with a chimney is illustrated by fig. 16. A tube is laid between the ceiling of the room and the floor above, one end of which terminates in the chimney, and the other in the middle of the ceiling of the room. In this case, the exhaustion is facilitated by the chandelier, which is suspended below the opening, the heat of the lamps contributing to increase the current of air through the ventilating tube. The tube can be commanded by a valve in any part of its course, and the aperture in the ceiling completely concealed from view by ornamental work. It is evident that the tube which connects the chimney with the room to be ventilated, may be of almost any length, provided it is perfectly air-tight at the sides.

This principle of ventilation may be applied in a great variety of modes, and in almost any situation. There are many houses and rooms, however, warmed by stoves, in which it may appear impossible to find a proper place, or sufficient space, for an aperture directly into the flue. Such is the case particularly in the tenements generally occupied by the poor of cities, where the low ceilings and narrow spaces leave too little room for cutting an opening, in addition to the one required for the stove-pipe. To obviate the difficulties presented in these cases, at the same time to obtain all the benefits of the smoke-flue for ventilation of the apartment, the plan represented in fig. 17 is recommended.

A stove-pipe is in fact a flue, and acts upon the same principle as a brick chimney, and may therefore be adapted to the ventilation of the room in which it is placed, in a manner similar to that described and illustrated by fig. 14. If the horizontal section of pipe (fig. 17) is made to project a short distance so as to form a T, and the end distant from the chimney is left open, a current of air will be observed to set into the pipe through the opening (as indicated by the arrow) as long as the pipe, or the chimney with which it is connected, is of an elevated temperature.

To render this method effective, however, care must be taken always to have the *ventilating portion* of the pipe, of a *larger diameter* than the other parts. The necessity for this will be understood, when it is remem-

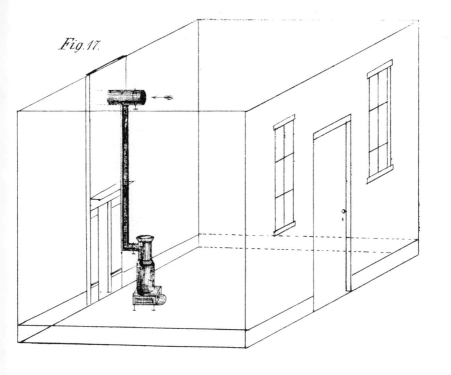

Fig. 17.

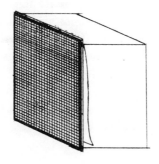

Fig. 18.

bered that stovepipes are generally of so small dimensions, that they are sufficient only for the gases which are required to be carried off from the fire; hence, to enable them to receive the volume of atmospheric air, necessary to be carried off for the purpose of ventilation, an increased capacity of pipe is required. For the same reason, the chimney-flue must have a capacity sufficient for all the air and gases sent into it.

The question will naturally arise, is there not great danger of a regurgitation in the flue or pipe, whereby smoke, or soot, or even sparks of fire, may be driven back into the apartment? and if so, how is it to be prevented?

To obviate this difficulty (which, however, can scarcely occur in a chimney of proper construction, when heated), two methods may be employed. One is, by placing a valve or register in the aperture of the flue or pipe, so arranged as to be readily closed and opened by hand. Another method of simple construction and having the advantage of being *self-acting*, has been suggested by an English writer, Dr. Arnott. It is represented by fig. 18, and consists merely of a light frame-work of tin or iron, the front of which is faced with a perforated zinc plate, or, what is better, wire-gauze. Behind the gauze is suspended, by its upper edge, a light curtain of some impervious material, which will be carried inward by the current of air as it passes into the chimney through the gauze, but which, whenever the air in the chimney regurgitates, falls, and is driven against the gauze, and thus closes the aperture against the egress of smoke or other gases. This little apparatus may be so made as to be slipped into the aperture in the flue, or the open end of the stovepipe. It is easily removed to be cleansed or repaired, should it ever be required, and may be made ornamental.

19

In fig. 19 will be found a further illustration of the effect of connecting the flue of the chimney with the apartment by means of a tube placed *behind the cornice*, all round the room, and opening into the latter at several points through the ornamental work of the cornice. The removal of the impure air of the room is not effected any more rapidly by this method; but there is an advantage in having a large number of points for its exit, while this arrangement may be practised sometimes when any other, equally good, might be inconvenient or impossible. (The dotted lines, representing the direction of the currents of air, should have been more diffused toward the entire cornice, and not so much concentrated to the main point of exit; — a correction which the reader will readily make in imagination.)

Fig. 20 illustrates the same principle again; in this case, the ventilating tube opens in the middle of the ceiling. The direction of the currents in this case, even of the cooler air entering by the doors and windows, is decidedly different from that represented in fig. 12, in which case the draught of the fire, in addition to the natural weight of the air, causes it to fall more or less directly to the floor.

In figure 22, may be seen another illustration of the effect of a ventilation, such as has been described, by an opening made directly into the chimney-flue, or, as in the drawing, into a separate ventilating shaft, adjacent to, and receiving heat from. the chimney. In this case, the mouth of the chimney and the ventilating aperture aid each other in exhausting the room of its air, which here finds itself replenished from the doors and windows, there being no regular apertures for the supply of pure air. Exhaustion by these methods, however, will be found sufficient, in any ordinary dwelling, not over-crowded, to maintain a degree of purity of

Fig 19.

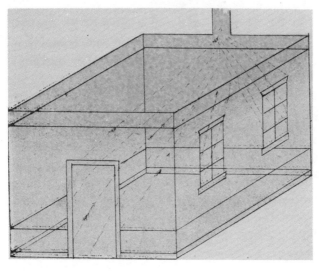

Fig. 20.

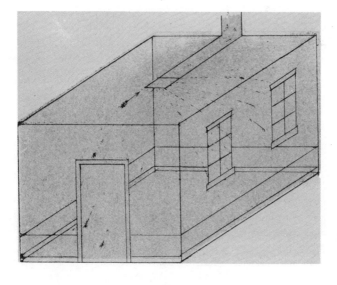

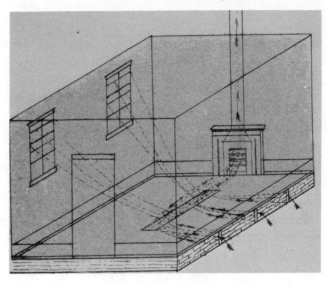

Fig. 21.

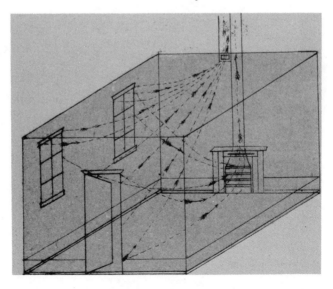

Fig. 22.

atmosphere sufficient for health, and to which the most luxuriously as well as the most meanly furnished houses are entire strangers, without it or some other equally effective method.

Fig. 21 is intended to show the principle of a plan suggested by Joseph Curtis, of New York, for the supply of fresh air in a more regular and systematic manner, and the removal of the impure air, which is applicable to any kind of house, but is more particularly adapted to schools, hospitals, and buildings of that character. The plan is as follows: beneath the floor, between the beams, an air-channel extends across the house, and through the walls at each side. This channel is connected with the apartment by an opening in the floor. At each end of the air-channel is a valve, by which it may be completely closed at pleasure. It will be seen, that if the channel has an east and west direction, for example, when the wind blows against the east side of the house, if the eastern valve is open and the western valve is closed, a stream of fresh air will be forced into the apartment through the opening in the floor: then, if the windows of the *west* side are opened a little distance, the current of air *through the room* will be complete, and will carry the impure air along with it. During a westerly wind, the eastern valve should be closed, and the windows of the same side open. When all the circumstances are favorable, this is a most effective plan of ventilation. No cold air can enter through the open window, as that would be contrary to the pressure without, and the aperture in the floor may be by diffusion plates, or be allowed in cold weather to open under the stove, so that the fresh air, before being diffused through the room, may be warmed. By this method a room may be supplied with fresh air, and exhausted of its impure air, to a sufficient extent, when all the

necessary circumstances concur.   This concurrence may,
however, often fail : 1st, there may be no wind outside ;
2d, it may not blow in the right direction ; 3d, the teacher
or sexton, or whoever may be in charge, must make
frequent and accurate observations, and close and open
the proper valve and windows as the changes of wind
may require.   The absence of either of these contingen-
cies will prevent the consummation desired ; but when
they are all present, a pure atmosphere may be almost
certainly expected in the apartment.

The moving powers, besides the agency of heat, used
in ventilating, are numerous.   The principal are various
kinds of *fans*, *pumps*, and *bellows ;* the use of the fan-
blower being generally to supply the air, though it is
sometimes used for a contrary purpose, viz., to draw it
off.   A particular description of these would be inconsistent with the intended size and object of this work :
as for them, a power, such as steam or horse power, is
necessary to move the machinery, and full descriptions
of these are to be found in various works.*   The *fan*
was first introduced to general notice by Desaguliers,
in the ventilation of the British Houses of Parliament
and the navy.   Hales invented the *bellows*, or rather a
machine on the principle of the common bellows, which
was used in the navy, and only employed in pumping
air into ships.   Both these plans soon fell into disuse ;
but Dr. Reid has lately revived the fan system, and
improved it into one of the arrangements for ventilating
the new Houses of Parliament.

The fan-blower, when operated with a strong motive
power, is perhaps the most efficient means, for either
supplying or exhausting air, that can be employed.   In

* Vide Wyman's treatise, in which he describes the *fan, bellows, windsail, turncaps, cowls,* &c., and the particular cases in which each is
applicable.

all manufactories where there is a steam-engine, and in every steamboat and steamship, it can be added to the machinery already existing with very little cost; and the great volume of air which it is capable of driving in or drawing off, enables even a moderate-sized one to ventilate a great extent of space. Almost any school or public room, or even a number of dwellings, in the vicinity of a steam-engine, can be connected with it by tubes.

In the capitol at Albany, New York, may be seen an arrangement for heating and ventilating by the *plenum* method, and upon a plan somewhat similar to that recently introduced in the British House of Commons, the French chamber of peers, and other public buildings; and which has, more recently still, been adopted in several manufacturing establishments in New England. The plan is, therefore, not an untried experiment, and is substantially as follows:—

A steam-engine is provided, of sufficient power to drive a revolving fan of suitable dimensions to move with force and velocity a quantity of atmospheric air, sufficient to supply the inmates of the apartment to be warmed and ventilated. The atmosphere thus put in motion, is conducted through tubes enveloped in steam, of a temperature not exceeding 212° Fahrenheit, by which means it will imbibe a genial heat, and will not become burned or decomposed. When thus heated, the air is conducted into a mixing chamber of brick-work, say twenty feet square, and thence by tubes into the various apartments of the building to be heated and ventilated.

This method is purely the *plenum*, and is deficient in means for removing the air after being used; in consequence of which a decided feeling of *oppressiveness* is experienced, which free exhaust openings would materially relieve.

19*

CHAPTER XVII.

PRACTICAL REMARKS ON WARMING AND VENTILATION.

Mixed Method of Ventilation.—Natural Currents of Wind made available.
—Cowls; receiving and exhausting.—Passenger-Ships.—Only available
when the Wind blows; an unsafe dependence.—*Heat*, the only Power
capable of general Application.—Warm Flues.—Houses without Flues;
how may be supplied with them.—Mode of applying Heat.—Difficult
Point to be obtained in warming.—Common Fires.—Air-tight Stoves.—
Open Charcoal or Anthracite Fires.—Heating by Hot Water or Steam.—
Objections to it.—Effect of Red-Hot Surfaces.—The most Healthful Prin-
ciple of Warming.—Obstacles encountered by Furnaces in general.—
Requisites for a proper Warming Apparatus.—*Ventilating Furnace* de-
scribed.—Further Illustrations of Ventilation.—Explanation of Plates.—
Reflections on the Subject.

A COMBINATION of the plenum and vacuum movements, denominated the *mixed method* of ventilation (by
which is meant the introduction of fresh air into the
apartment, simultaneously with the withdrawal of the
impure air from it), being that which alone can insure
entire salubrity of atmosphere in any situation, it is
proper in this stage of our remarks to inquire what are
the plans best adapted to this end, in circumstances of
ordinary domiciliation. And as in cold seasons of the
year, it is necessary to have an atmosphere warmed to a
proper temperature, before it is introduced into an apartment, it is of the highest importance that the mode of
warming the air does not, in any degree, impair its
healthful properties.

So far as natural currents of wind may be depended
on, to ventilate rooms or buildings, the most efficient

method of supplying fresh, and removing the foul air, independent of windows, is to underlay the floors with one or more air-channels, running their whole length, one end terminating in flues, which ascend above the roof, in the side-walls. Each flue is to be surmounted by a *receiving cowl*, so that whenever the wind blows, a current of air will be forced down the flues into the air-channels, and into the apartments, through diffusing plates, placed in the floors, which plates form the upper sides of the air-channels. This constitutes the *plenum* part of the arrangement.

To complete the plan, other flues are made in the *opposite* wall of the house, and open into the apartments at the *ceilings*. The latter flues are surmounted at the roof with *exhausting cowls*.

The same current of wind which forces air into the apartment through the receiving cowl, will operate upon the exhausting cowl, and force it out ; and thus, under favorable circumstances, a volume of air more or less copious, must be made to pass through the apartment.

The arrangement above described must depend in a great degree upon the efficiency of the cowls, by which the flues in the walls are terminated, and, so far as experiment has enabled the question to be settled, the palm of superiority appears to be awarded to the exhausting cowl, invented by Jordan L. Mott.

The cuts on the next page represent both the receiving and exhausting cowls, made by Mott.

On examination of these figures, the reader will at once perceive that the same wind which operates upon the exhausting cowl to produce a vacuum, must also act upon the plenum cowl, to drive the air into its mouth. Whatever may be their relative position, one must receive, the other exhaust, the air.

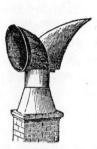 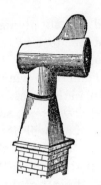

Plenum or receiving cowl, the open   Vacuum or exhausting cowl, open
mouth to the wind.   at both ends.

This method is now adopted in many of the passenger-vessels arriving in this country, under the act of Con-
gress of July, 1848, requiring their ventilation. The air-
channels, perforated at numerous points, are laid along
the floor of the steerage or cabin, connected at the after-
end with a tube which projects above the deck, and is
surmounted with a receiving cowl; at the forward end
of the steerage, another tube pierces the deck from the
ceiling, and is terminated with a vacuum cowl. Thus a
good ventilation may be had, even in stormy weather,
when the hatches are necessarily all closed, and battened
down ; in fact, the stronger the wind, the more abundant
must be the ventilation.

By this method, however, ventilation can only be obtained *when the wind blows.* It is true, its failure on this
account may not often occur, as a perfect calm very seldom happens, and is rarely of long duration; nevertheless, it is during a calm that ventilation is most needed,
and the uncertainty of its operation, at one time, perhaps, not operating at all, at another too powerfully,
makes it less satisfactory than is desirable for continually-
occupied rooms or workshops.

Under the circumstances in which this method of ventilation is generally employed, it is of course necessary

that the air be warmed, if warmed at all, in the apartment itself. The sources of heat must therefore be the usual ones of stoves of various kinds, or the common grate or fireplace, and when this plan of ventilation is effective, it makes but little difference how the heat is obtained, as the abundant supply of air, and the free removal of it after being used, must prevent or overcome any deterioration of its quality.

But, as before hinted, the wind is an unsafe dependence, and the operations of a ventilating arrangement which relies solely upon it, can not be regulated to suit all the changes of temperature, season, or number of people.

For all kinds of dwelling-houses, churches, school-houses, and public halls, except those in which *mechanical force* can be applied to the purposes of ventilation (in which case the fan-blower constitutes the most powerful and cheapest arrangement, for both supplying and exhausting air), *heat* is the only motive power, capable of general application. By its agency, a current of air may always certainly be established, and the only question for the builder or the occupant to consider, relates to the manner in which it can be most advantageously applied.

Whenever a flue capable of being warmed can be obtained, communicating with the room required to be ventilated, there is at once a means of removing the impure air, and the openings for the introduction of pure air, may be made where most convenient. The exhaustion of the air by the warm flue, must necessarily cause an ingress of fresh air to an equal amount.

In houses already built without flues, wooden troughs or channels may be made to answer the purpose; these should be made perfectly air-tight at the joints, and extend from the room to be ventilated, perpendicularly to the attic of the building, where they should terminate in iron or brick flues, to extend out through the roof, somewhat in the manner of a chimney. In the latter extension a small fire, of wood or coal, or even a lamp or gaslight, will often give sufficient heat to cause a draught strong enough to ventilate a large room.

When there is more than one room in a house to be ventilated by extemporaneous means, a flue such as those just described may be carried from each apartment, and all be concentrated into one brick or iron extension, the fire in which will cause a current through all the tubes opening into it, which will be strong in proportion to the degree of heat, and height of the chimney.

In this climate, where the vicissitudes of heat and cold are so great, the temperature of the air is an important consideration, and as cold is often almost immediate in its effects upon the constitution, it may be said to have received a due share of attention. Human ingenuity has always been busy in fortifying the body against cold, and death is often said to make his approach in the shape of a *cold draught* through a keyhole.

One of the most difficult points to be attained in warming, is to avoid these cold draughts (as they are less tolerable to many than positive and uniform coldness), or, in other words, to equalize the temperature in every part of the room, which can not be done when the doors and windows are open, or even when they are shut, unless the latter are double. When warm air is thrown into a room, it should emerge at as many apertures as possible, and if the air is warmed by a stove, or otherwise, it should be carried off, when once breathed, by suitable openings, or apparatus, at the ceiling; while the fresh air should be admitted in like quantity, and with like velocity.

Common fires in fireplaces or grates, though they do

not heat the air so uniformly or economically, are more wholesome than the ordinary kind of stoves, because they draw off the air of the apartment more copiously and rapidly. Stoves (especially when heated to redness) considerably deteriorate the air, and unfit it for healthy respiration, principally because they have so little draught, and cause so little renewal of the atmosphere. What are called *air-tight* stoves, warm very economically, but at the entire expense of ventilation, and, consequently, of health. These should never be employed unless there is a direct and positive means of ventilation.

The practice of placing an open vessel containing burning anthracite or charcoal, in a close chamber, to heat the air, is either positively criminal, or at best evinces the grossest ignorance. From the latter substance, pure carbonic acid gas, in great quantities, and from the former, carbonic oxide, which is equally deleterious, are given off.

In heating by steam or hot water, the boiler may be detached considerably from the building or apartment intended to be warmed, into which the steam or water is conveyed through iron pipes, and thus the danger of fire is materially lessened. This plan is attended with great outlay of money and expenditure of fuel, and many precautions are required in managing the steam-pipes. The water is liable to continue cold a long time, in the pipes occupying places in the room most distant from the boiler; but they have the advantage when once heated, of remaining so.

With reference to ventilation, this mode of warming is liable to the same objection as air-tight stoves—*there being no air introduced into the apartment with the heat.*

There are several buildings warmed in this manner in New York city, the Tract-house, in Nassau street, for example, and though there is no danger of the air being

injured by the heat (the temperature of the radiating surface not being above 212 degrees), yet there being no
ventilation, the gases of respiration become concentrated
in the several apartments, without chance of escape.

In those arrangements in which heat is imparted from
red-hot surfaces, the air is said to be *burned* or *scorched*,
and has a *close, sulphurous* smell. Though this description is vague, and the *principle* on which the air is made
unwholesome not yet satisfactorily explained, it is a fact
that persons who respire such air complain of "headache, giddiness, stupor," &c.

*Undoubtedly the most healthful principle upon which
artificial warmth for houses is to be obtained, is by warming the air before it reaches the apartment, and then forcing it, or drawing it in, in copious quantities.*—Besides
being the most healthful, *when properly adapted to its
purpose,* this is believed to be also the most economical
principle of securing a proper temperature, and for the
latter consideration it is, as it would appear, chiefly, that
so much attention has been given to the construction of
hot air furnaces, and the great diversity of forms which
have emanated from the office of the Commissioner of
Patents.

That economy, and not health, has been the principal
motive of the inventors of this kind of apparatus for the
exercise of their ingenuity, is very apparent from the utter regardlessness of the preservation of the healthful
properties of the air thrown into the apartment, exhibited
in the construction of most of the furnaces now in vogue.
It is this fact that has undoubtedly deterred, and still
continues to deter, many, from the introduction of this
mode of warming into their houses; the principles upon
which nearly all the furnaces, now generally used, are
constructed and located, being unphilosophical, destructive of material, and producing unnecessary loss of ca-

loric, and consequent waste of fuel, without any attention whatever to the subject of ventilation.

To illustrate these remarks, a few facts will suffice, to which the attention of those who already have, or expect to have, hot-air furnaces in their dwellings or other houses, should be directed.

1st. Few, if any, of the heaters now in general use, are able to impart a sufficient temperature to the air to warm the area of an ordinary dwelling, without raising the iron of the furnace to a *red heat*, whereby, as before remarked, the healthful properties of the air are greatly impaired.

2d. The areas of the hot-air chambers are so small, and the openings into and from them so contracted, that the air, being unable to circulate freely through them, is detained in close proximity to the hot iron surface too long, and is then thrown into the apartment in too small quantities. When this is the case, the temperature of the air must necessarily be very high, in order to warm the apartment sufficiently; whereas a large bulk of air freely diffused through a room, will impart warmth enough, though its own temperature may be but slightly raised.

These constitute the most prominent evils, so far as the internal arrangement of the furnace is concerned. But another, and perhaps more serious evil still, is to be found, in some instances, in

3d. The location of the furnace, and the source from which it derives the air to be warmed. The furnace must be placed in the lowest room or cellar of the building, that the warm air may freely ascend; but unless proper arrangements are made to receive a supply of air from the outside of the building, the atmosphere of the house itself will be drawn into the furnace-chamber, there be heated, be returned to the house, be drawn back again to the furnace, and thus be made to traverse

20

the circle of the house and the furnace, as long as the latter is in operation.

That such an arrangement as this should for a single day be permitted, is as strange as it is true, and reflects no more discredit upon the inventor or builder of the furnace, than upon the proprietor of the tenement who admits it, and breathes, or permits others to breathe, in continuous succession, the air thus warmed. Less excusable still was it, in the government of one of the largest and most flourishing female seminaries of the intelligent city of New York, that three large heaters were thus arranged, by which the air of the apartments to be warmed, was drawn almost in direct lines to the furnaces, there heated by red-hot iron surfaces, and then returned through the hot-air pipes, to the school-rooms, where it again passed through the lungs of the pupils, to be again drawn down to the furnaces, and was thus made to flow perpetually in the same currents, the whole atmosphere of the house being, the while, offensive and poisonous. This arrangement was blindly continued several winters, before its evils were pointed out, after which an improvement in the source of the air was effected.

The same vicious arrangement may be found in some of our churches, and other buildings, both public and private.

Until very recently, the attention of no truly philosophical mind, and but little liberality of means, in this country at least, appear to have been directed to the construction and arrangement of such an apparatus for warming, as, while meeting the proper requirements of economy of fuel, should compass the *principal* end to which these means ought always to be directed, viz., the constant maintenance of a pure atmosphere within the building with which the apparatus is connected. This end, however, is now within the reach of all who are able to command it, at the same time that the consideration of economy is equally well sustained.

To Arnott and Reid, in England, and Curtis and Bull, of our own country, are we indebted for the application of much intelligent thought, and sound principles of philosophy, to the arrangement of apparatuses specially devoted to the purposes of warming and ventilation.

In continuation of the design of this and the preceding chapter, of presenting ideas of the arrangements best and most easily adapted to these ends, in the majority of buildings, with the least cost and greatest efficiency, the following description is given of the plan arranged by James H. Bull, of New York, as it is seen in operation in several public and private buildings. It combines economy of fuel and salubrity of atmosphere, with moderation of temperature and copiousness of volume, *and a direct and positive ventilation*, in such a manner and sufficiency as scarcely to leave anything to be desired, except what can only be obtained by a much heavier outlay of money.

To comprehend fully the merits of this arrangement, it will be necessary to understand what is required of a hot-air furnace, and the difficulties to be overcome by it.

The advantages of a properly-constructed hot-air furnace, over other modes of imparting heat to rooms and tenements, are, *first*, the warming of a large area (one large room or several small rooms) by one fire ; in other words, economy of fuel and labor ; *second*, the introduction into the apartments, of a continuous supply of fresh air, properly warmed ; and *third*, the removal of the old air as rapidly as possible.

These being the ends necessary to be secured, it

follows that that arrangement is to be preferred by which they are the most fully and readily accomplished.

The greater the area warmed by a given amount of fuel and in a given time — the more copious the supply of fresh air, and the more genial its temperature — and the more complete and efficient the removal of the old air — in these will consist the superiority of any particular plan or apparatus, for warming and ventilation.

To obtain a large radiating surface, which shall receive its heat directly from the fire, is a very desirable point: 1st, because the greatest amount of heat will then be imparted to the air, and more rapidly; 2d, because the air may then be warmed without the furnace being raised to a red heat. The smoke-flue should be regarded only as a secondary source of radiation, instead of a primary one, as in most of the furnaces now constructed.

The principal objection to the present general arrangement of hot-air furnaces, is the *obstacles met with in introducing the warm air into an apartment.* The air in a furnace-chamber having a tendency to rise, just as smoke rises in a flue, a part of it will enter and occupy any other space, which may be in connexion with the air-chamber; and cold air being admitted into the latter, its greater weight will continue to press the heated air upward. But if the apartment to be heated is *close and tight,* it is evident that the air it already contains will resist the entrance of any additional quantity; being already full, it will contain no more; the pressure of the heated air may overcome the resistance to a small, but it will be a very small, extent.

This may be illustrated by making the attempt to blow into a tight bottle, through its mouth; the resistance is sufficient to overcome the most powerful effort of the lungs.

By many it is supposed that the crevices in the doors and windows, and other apertures, will allow the air to go out of the room, and thus enable the air from the furnace to find its way into it.   This may be true to a certain extent, but not to the degree generally supposed, for very often the wind outside is pressing *in* at the same crevices, thus increasing the resistance to the current of hot air; and at any rate, these apertures are uncertain, very irregular, and afford no surety for the escape of the air of the room.

But if we suppose the apartment which is to be heated, is too tight to admit air through these crevices (which it will be if the carpenter has done justice to the work), it is manifest that the attempt to force air in, under the ordinary pressure of a furnace, can be only partially successful, and that what air does find its way in, will rise at once to the ceiling, be confined for a long time there, and at that part of the room at which it entered, and can not find its way *through* the room, except by the currents caused by changes of temperature, which are necessarily very slow.

The obstacles thus preventing the diffusion of the air from the furnace, also interfere with the diffusion of the heat, for the air, which is the vehicle of the heat into the room, being unable to carry it further than the immediate vicinity of its point of entrance, the heat itself must also necessarily find its way very slowly through the apartment.   The latter objection amounts, principally, to a loss of time in warming, and consequently involves a great waste of fuel, as a larger amount must be consumed to supply a sufficiency of heated air; while it is obvious, that if a great volume of air heated to a lower temperature. could, by any means, be thrown into the room, but especially if the current thus introduced can be made to pass more or less quickly *through* the room,

20*

there will be a proportionate economy of time, fuel, and comfort.

But another consideration of far greater importance than those of economy of time and fuel, is *economy of health ;* and in the selection of a means of warming, with reference to this end, the *first consideration* should be, *a large volume of air, raised to a moderate temperature* forced or drawn quickly through the room ; and *the next* is, the rapid removal of all the products of respiration, perspiration, combustion, &c. When these points are secured, the consideration of economy is also obtained, for the means which must be used to obtain the first consideration, and to avoid their opposites, are such as must necessarily be followed by the last.

With the rapid distribution of the warm air from the furnace, through the apartment, the heat is carried along and diffused with it.

That apparatus, therefore, which throws into an apartment the largest amount of air — which warms it sufficiently without a red-hot surface — which diffuses it most rapidly and directly through the room — which furnishes a means of removing the foul air — and which does not require the evaporation of a large amount of water to restore the moisture to the air, of which an intense heat has deprived it — that furnace which accomplishes these objects most readily, is entitled to the first regard, on account of both its healthful and economical properties.

There are some hot-air furnaces which have attained some of these ends, but as yet there has appeared but one arrangement which successfully accomplishes them all, and which alone is therefore justly entitled to the name of a *ventilating furnace.* Of that one, planned and put in successful operation, within the past year (1848), by Mr. Bull, a brief description will be here given.

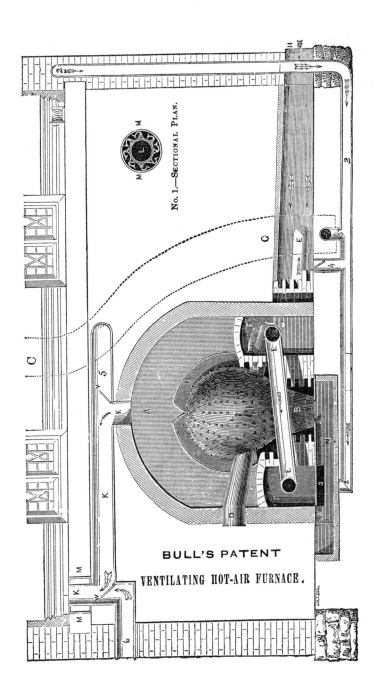

No. 1.—Sectional Plan.

BULL'S PATENT
VENTILATING HOT-AIR FURNACE.

SECTIONAL DRAWING.

[The *letters* refer to the warming part of the apparatus, the *figures* to the ventilating part.]

A, A. A. Hot-air chamber of brick.

B. Fire-pot, lined with soapstone or fire-brick.

C. Spherical fire-chamber, studded with radiating points.

D. Feed-flue.

E, E, E. Smoke-pipe, emerging from the fire-chamber, just above the fire, and conducted obliquely downward around the fire-pot, and passing (as indicated by arrows) through

F, F. A separate brick channel, built inside the air-chamber, at its base. The smoke-pipe finally enters

G, G. The chimney of the house.

H. Cold-air entrance.

I, I. Heat radiators, or *distributors,* of sheet-iron.

K, K. Hot-air discharge-pipe.

L. Register, in the floor of the apartment.

M, M. Cast-iron water-tank, surrounding the end of the hot-air pipe.

N. Ash-pit.

1. Opening of the ventilating duct, at the opposite side of the room, from the hot-air register.

2, 2, 2. Ventilating duct, terminating at the ash-pit, N, through which the foul air is drawn in by the fire, and consumed.

3. Branch ventilating duct, governed by a valve, and entering directly into the smoke-flue.

4, Branch duct, with a valve. supplying the hot-air chamber, A, with air from the apartment to be ventilated ; to be used only for summer ventilation.

5. Branch pipe, for discharging heated air from the hot-air chamber, A, into the chimney, when the valve V is open.

6. Pipe for replenishing the apartment with cold air from out-doors, when the valve W is perpendicular.

In the annexed drawing of the *ground plan* (No. 2), the arrangement of the smoke-pipe, and cold-air flue, is more distinctly shown, the same reference letters being used as in the sectional view ; E, E, E, being the smoke-pipe, passing out from C, the fire-chamber, through the separate brick channel F, F, F, and terminating in G, the chimney. The arrows *inside* the smoke-pipe indicate the direction which the smoke takes, while other arrows, *outside* the smoke-pipe, indicate the course of the fresh cold air from without.

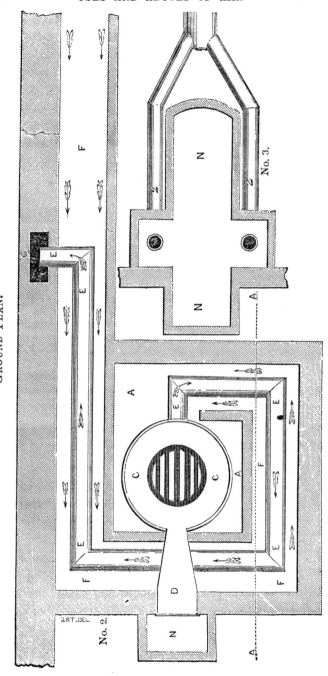

BULL'S PATENT VENTILATING HOT-AIR FURNACE.

Ground Plan.

In drawing No. 3, is represented the manner in which the foul-air ducts, 2, 2, open into the ash-pit, N, N. The openings are directly under the grate of the fire-pot, and so guarded as to prevent ashes and cinders from falling into them.

The points wherein the arrangements of this furnace, regarded merely as a heater, appear superior to others, are,

First. The manner in which the cold external air is made to enter the hot-air chamber. It enters through the same channel by which the smoke-pipe goes out, and as it passes by the latter, receives the heat from it, whereby it is considerably raised in temperature, before it enters the main air-chamber itself. A great amount of caloric, therefore, which would otherwise be (and is by any other plan) lost by being sent into the chimney-flue, is thus preserved and imparted to the fresh air. So effectual is this arrangement, that even where the fire is brisk, the end of the smoke-pipe, as it enters the chimney, is barely warm to the hand.

Second. The mode by which the direct heat of the spherical radiator is imparted to the air in the hot-air chamber. The greater the amount of radiating surface, the more rapidly will the air be heated. I I are screens of sheet-iron, placed about midway between the heater and the brick walls of the chamber. These are so arranged that the air flows freely among them, while they intercept the rays of heat, and prevent them, in a great measure, from falling upon, and being absorbed by, the brick-work ; at the same time, they act as *distributors* of the heat to the air as it passes through the air-chamber. In all other furnaces hitherto observed, the smoke-pipe is taken off from the heater, at the top, and is freely exposed in the air-chamber itself, its surface being relied upon mainly for radiating heat to the air around it. It is, however, very doubtful whether more heat is not imparted to, than is received from, the pipe, by the air in the chamber, for it will be perceived that as the fresh air enters the air-chamber, at its lowest part, it flows against the hottest part of the heater, *first*, where it immediately gets highly heated, and after that, rises against the smoke-pipe, which must be cooler than the heater itself, and therefore cooler than the air surrounding it. Does not the smoke-pipe, therefore, receive caloric from the air, instead of imparting caloric to it? By the arrangement adopted by Mr. Bull, the smoke-pipe imparts all its caloric to the fresh air, except so much as is necessary to maintain a draught in the chimney-flue.

The space which is occupied by the smoke-pipe, in other furnaces, from which heat is falsely supposed to be given off is occupied, in the plan here described, by the large screens I I, which add largely to the radiating surface, and therefore heat the air more rapidly.

But it is as an apparatus for ventilation, that Mr. Bull's patent claims our especial notice. It will be observed, in the *first* place, *that as long as the fire burns*, or as long as the apparatus or the chimney-flue is warm, there must be a stream of air drawn off from the room above, carried off through the fire, into the chimney, and discharged through the latter into the open air.

Secondly, the difficulties which were noted on page 232 as existing in the way of forcing the air from a furnace into a room, are entirely removed by Mr. Bull's arrangement; for not only is there a vent-hole for the *escape* of air from one side of the room, as the warm air is forced in at the other side, but a current, more or less strong, is *drawn* through the vent-hole, by the burning of the fire below. A partial vacuum is thus created in the room above, which is most easily supplied through the register at the opposite side, in consequence of which, while the foul air is removed, a more copious supply of fresh, warm air, is introduced.

This leads us to notice the *third* important consideration, viz., the more rapid distribution of the air *through* the room, carrying with it the heat, and the consequent saving of time and fuel, in warming the apartment.

There is yet one other idea of much value embraced in this apparatus, in which others are deficient. When a building or room, warmed by a furnace of ordinary construction, becomes over-heated, the register through which the heat is supplied must be closed, but in doing so, not only the heat, but likewise the air is shut out, and whatever advantage was derived from the small volume of air which forced its way in, is now entirely lost, and during the time required to cool down the surplus heat of the room, impurities are accumulating in the atmosphere.

But should it be necessary at any time, to reduce the temperature of a room warmed by the furnace above described, it may be done more rapidly, and without cutting off the supply of air, by simply raising the valve W, by which a current of cold external air is admitted, combined, at will, with the warm air from the furnace. The exhaustion from the opposite side of the room, draws in an equal amount of air, warm or cold, or of mixed temperature, according as the valve is opened fully or partially.

As described thus far, this arrangement is applied to warming and ventilating — operations which are required to be performed together only in cold weather. The inventor's ingenuity, however, has not stopped here, but by a simple contrivance, the furnace is adapted also to ventilation without warming, a great desideratum not only in summer (when purity of air may be best maintained by open doors and windows), but at other sea-

21

sons, when the weather is too cool for open windows, and
yet too warm for fires, but when ventilation is as much
needed as ever. It is effected in the following manner :—

A small fire kindled in the heater, will cause a draught
down through the ventilating duct, 2, 2, to supply the
combustion. The air in the hot-air chamber will be
warmed and rarified, but instead of being allowed to
pass into the apartment at K, the valve W is drawn up
perpendicularly, while the valve V is thrown open wide,
and the heated air then escapes through the pipe 5, into
the chimney-flue. To increase the ventilation, the valve
at H being closed, the valve in the branch pipe 4 is
opened, by which a current of air will be drawn in to
the hot-air chamber, to go through it up the chimney,
and thus the current through 1 and 2, is largely increased. The exhaustion thus produced from one side
of the room, causes an equal influx of fresh air through
the open pipe 6, at the opposite side.

It is neither recommended nor intended that the means
of ventilation presented by this arrangement, should su-
persede other methods, which, in many situations, may
be more easily and economically put in practice. Nor,
in fact, should it be solely relied on, under general circumstances ; but as an improvement upon the usual
methods of warming, and especially as furnishing a
means of ventilation, with very little additional expense,
this arrangement deserves earnest consideration.

It is in the building of a house that ventilating arrangements may be introduced with the least cost, and greatest facility. So far as the introduction of ventilating-
flues in the walls, or of air-channels under the floors of
houses of any kind, is concerned, not only may they be
introduced with very little cost, but in very many instances houses may be erected at less cost with them, than
without them. In buildings whose walls are of brick or

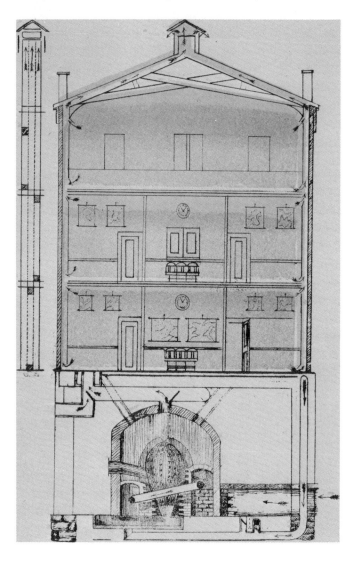

Fig. 24.   Fig. 23.

stone, the introduction of a flue, which is merley *a vacancy of material*, there may be a sufficient saving of material and labor, to pay for all that may be requisite to complete the plan of ventilation. This economical view of the subject, it is hoped, will operate as an inducement upon each one who builds a house hereafter, to cause ventilating flues to be left in the walls, so that should the first proprietor be so indifferent to his own comfort and that of others, as to permit foul air to accumulate in it, his heirs and successors, who may have a better appreciation of the importance and comfort of a wholesome atmosphere, may be able to obtain it, without any further cost or trouble, than merely to connect the flues with the apartments.

Having laid down, in the preceding pages, some of the general principles upon which the ventilation of buildings is to be effected, it remains now only to state more particularly how these principles are to be reduced to practice, and for this purpose, the universal language of pictures will be further resorted to.

In fig. 23 is seen a sectional representation of a school-house, three stories in height, ventilated by the double method of flues in the walls, concentrated in the cupola or ejector on the roof, aided by the ventilating furnace in the cellar. The flues, or *venti-ducts*, as they are properly called, numbering at least one for each room, are connected with the apartments by two apertures in each, one near the ceiling, the other near the floor, either of which may be opened at pleasure. The fresh warm air in winter, proceeding from the furnace below, being thrown into the apartment at one side, the upper orifice of the venti-duct on the opposite side is closed, and the lower one opened. The warm air emerging from the register, is more or less rapidly drawn through the room, and when the desirable temperature has been obtained, and the pupils have assembled, the lower orifice is closed and the upper one opened. The impurities which are then generated, are more directly carried off.

Fig. 24 represents a lateral section of the venti-ducts or foul air-flues, showing the manner in which they are arranged and carried up separately from the floor of each room, until they discharge into the common ejector.

The venti-ducts are here represented as united together in the attic, under a cupola with side-openings, and arranged in such a manner that the wind will force the foul air out. Or the venti-ducts may be concentrated in one, terminating in a chimney, as described at page 226, in which a small fire may be kept during school hours.

The reader will not fail to compare the atmosphere of this house, as represented, with that of the school-house depicted in fig. 6.

In fig. 25 is a representation of the state of the atmosphere, during the progress of the service, in a non-ventilated church, the doors and windows being closed, and the lamps lighted.

Fig. 26 represents the condition of the atmosphere of the same church, after the introduction of ventilating arrangements (other circumstances being the same). The tower, or spire, is made to act as well for the introduction of fresh air, as for the removal of the impure air, and for both purposes it affords superior facilities. (In all cases the fresh air should be drawn from the highest possible portion of the building, as the higher the source, the further removed from the soil and less mingled with its emanations and impurities will it be.) In the figure, the fresh air is represented as introduced near the base of the tower, from which a long arrow indicates its descent below the main floor of the church. Having been warmed, or not, as circumstances require,

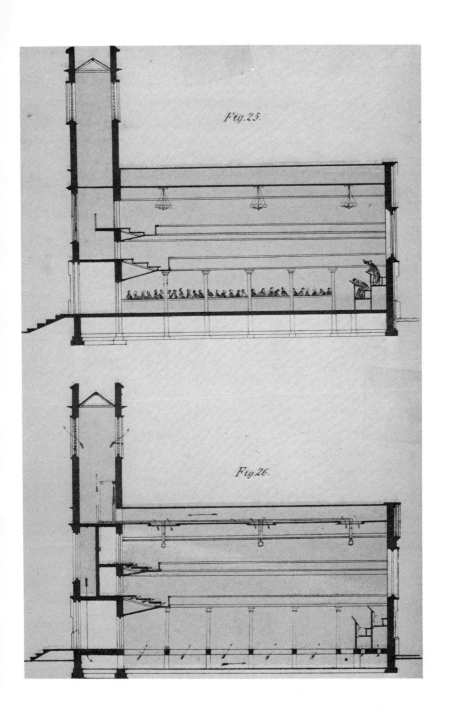

Fig.25.

Fig.26.

Fig. 27.

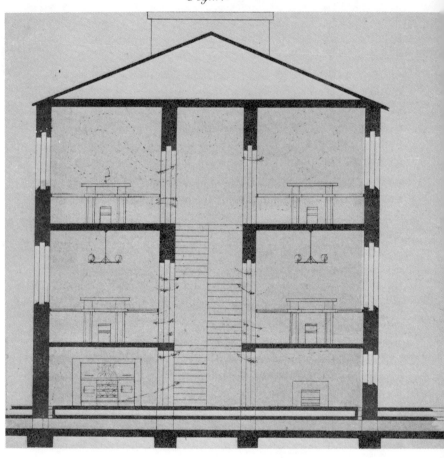

it is made to ascend through numerous openings in the floor, and is diffused through the entire body of the church, and finds its way out through apertures in the ceiling, immediately over the lamps, which, when burning, aid its progress very much. The products of respiration and combustion are received into a foul-air channel, which lies along over the ceiling in the attic, and is connected, by a special opening, with the upper part of the spire, through which, ultimately, the foul air escapes, aided by such an arrangement of windows or cowls, or combustion, as may be best adapted to the circumstances of the case.

At the point of union between the spire and the foul-air channel, a valve is placed, which is commanded from below by a cord and pulley (see figure); by means of this, the amount of discharge is regulated; being opened during service, and closed in the intervals, to prevent the unnecessary escape of heat.

In fig. 27 is an illustration of the progress of air in a house where the fittings render it almost entirely air-tight. It is filled with a vitiated atmosphere from products of respiration and combustion, scullery, water-closets, drains, back smoke, dust of carpets, &c. The rooms in the upper story afford the principal supply of fresh air by the chimneys, or such as are not in use, no other source being open. The great consumption of the kitchen enables it to draw largely from the passage, which again receives its supply from the rooms above. While these more general movements proceed in the manner indicated by the arrows, local currents are developed in other apartments by lamps and fireplaces, as well as by individuals respiring the vitiated air, indicated by dotted lines.

In fig. 28 is represented the same house, after having undergone some alterations, and the principal evils cor-

21*

rected by the introduction of a copious supply of fresh air (warmed in winter) into the stair-case, and passages, and the removal of the vitiated air from all the apartments, lamps, and drains. In cold weather, a Bull's furnace, or some equivalent apparatus, is placed in the lower central part of the house, and air is allowed to flow in so freely, that it is continually flooded with a warm atmosphere, tending, from its warmth, to escape upward, wherever an aperture is permitted. Communications are established between the passage and each apartment. By valves and appropriate channels, as have been described in the previous pages, the admission to, and discharge from, each apartment, are regulated. All the discharges and venti-ducts unite in a general foul-air chamber under the roof, which communicates with the open air by such an arrangement as is best adapted to the circumstances of the case; either a heated flue, an arrangement of windows, or properly-located exhausting cowls. The general discharge of foul air, is also regulated by a large valve in the foul-air chamber.

To insure, as much as possible, the avoidance of any foul gases from private drains, these should be trapped in the most careful manner, and a ventilating flue, if possible, be so arranged as to receive all the products which might otherwise be discharged into the room.

CONCLUDING REFLECTIONS.

The foregoing pages greatly outnumber their original estimate ; the apology, if one is needed, is to be found in the fact, that the subject belongs to a class, whose characteristic is, an interest increasing with the thought bestowed upon it. As the presence of the atmosphere, in its bountiful abundance and self-maintaining purity, when left to the working of its own natural laws, is universal, so may it be said, that the illustrations of its evil

Fig. 28.

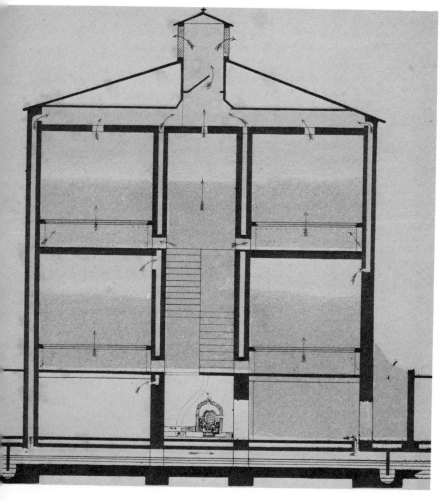

effects, when those laws are interfered with, and its natural freedom restrained, are everywhere to be found, and continually recurring.

It is no less true of the laws instituted to preserve the wholesomeness of the atmosphere, than of those relating to diet, or any other branch of physiology, that their violation is certain to be followed by punishment.

God has so plainly written these laws upon all his works, but especially upon that branch of them herein considered, that he who runs may read; nothing but the blindness of ignorance and of obstinate prejudice, can prevent their being seen.

If there is a responsibility resting upon intelligent creatures, in reference to obedience to the laws of Providence; if in proportion to our advancement in knowledge, that responsibility is made heavier and plainer; if the press, the steam-engine, and the telegraph, have many-fold increased the facilities and comforts of life, and brought us rapidly nearer to the glorious consummation of its great end, the enjoyment of existence in its purest form; what shall we answer to the charge of neglect of the plainest dictates of nature and of common sense, manifested by the continual violation of their laws, in regard to the great ocean of air in which we are immersed.

By rejecting the means presented to us for the preservation and prolongation of our lives, are we not as justly chargeable with suicide, as he who strangles himself with a cord? or is taking poison into the lungs, any more venial than taking it into the stomach? And when we reflect that a large proportion of the diseases of mankind are clearly traceable to atmospheric causes, and that those causes are, in a vast majority of cases, certainly and easily removable and preventible, how can we escape the condemnation which attaches to their continuance?

Especially is this condemnation deserved, when considered in comparison with that which follows the violation of many other laws of health. There is some apology for the drunkard and the gourmand; they have natural appetites for food and drink, which have obtained the mastery over their feeble wills, while the pleasures of the cup and table, entice increasingly with the loss of mental strength. But there is no such thing as appetite for foul air; we have no pleasure in it; no such idea can be pleaded in extenuation of the crime (for it is no less) of inhaling a substance well known to be a poison, when it is just as easy to avoid it.

To the educated, who can understand and appreciate the inestimable value of pure air, and to the rich, who are able to obtain, not only the necessities and comforts, but also the superfluities and extravagances of life, these remarks apply in all their force. But there are others, constituting the larger portion of mankind, in civilized life at least, who, from poverty, are compelled to crowd themselves into narrow domicils, or who, through ignorance, never reflect upon, and can not comprehend, the true relations of the atmosphere to their happiness and health. For their neglect of this important subject, there is some excuse; though conscious of suffering, of which they would gladly rid themselves, they know neither the cause nor the remedy, and it were as easy to count the sands of the seashore, as to estimate the lives which have been sacrificed upon this one altar in the great temple of ignorance and poverty.

Upon whom, then, rests the blame connected with this state of things? Certainly upon those who build and own the tenements of the poor. A just appreciation and regard of the wants of those, whose pittances of rent swell the great tide which flows into the landlords' coffers, would teach them to consider a pure atmosphere within the house, as necessary to make it tenantable as a tight roof. And it is for him whose buildings are occupied by the poor, who can not *command* a proper system of ventilation in their narrow quarters, to consider well and earnestly the duty he owes to his tenants, and provide them with a healthful atmosphere. There can not be a reasonable doubt, that were all the tenements occupied by the laboring classes, at once and thoroughly ventilated, the very small outlay required for the purpose, would be soon returned a hundred-fold, in the saving of health, life, and morals, and in a great diminution of the expenses incurred for the support of charitable institutions.

To those who have in charge the care and instruction of the rising generation — the future fathers and mothers of men — this subject commends itself with an interest surpassing that of any other. Nothing can more convincingly establish the belief of the existence of something essentially and vitally wrong in the habits and circumstances of civilized life, than the appalling fact, that one fourth of all who are born, die before reaching the fifth year, and that one half the deaths of mankind occur under the twentieth year.

Let those who have these things in charge, answer to their own consciences how they have discharged their duty, in supplying to the young, the responsibility of whose lives and education they have assumed — A PURE ATMOSPHERE, THE FIRST REQUISITE FOR HEALTHY BODIES AND SOUND MINDS.

THE END.

CONTENTS.

CHAPTER VII.

CHAPTER VIII.

CHAPTER IX.

CHAPTER X.

CHAPTER XI.

CHAPTER XII.

CHAPTER XIII.

CHAPTER XIV.

CHAPTER XV.

CHAPTER XVI.

CHAPTER XVII.